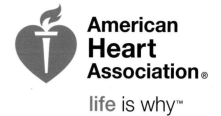

American
Heart
Association®

life is why™

Heartsaver®

PEDIATRIC FIRST AID CPR AED

STUDENT WORKBOOK

ISBN 978-1-61669-425-8
Printed in the United States of America
First American Heart Association Printing September 2016
10 9

Acknowledgments

The American Heart Association thanks the following people for their contributions to the development of this workbook: Jeff A. Woodin, NREMT-P; Mary Fran Hazinski, RN, MSN; Robert Lee Hanna; Kostas Alibertis, CCEMT-P; Jeanette Previdi, MPH, BSN, RN-BC; Mark Terry, MPA, NREMT-P; Moira Muldoon; Brenda Schoolfield; and the AHA Heartsaver Project Team.

 To find out about any updates or corrections to this text, visit **www.heart.org/cpr**, navigate to the page for this course, and click on "Updates."

Contents

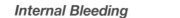

life is why.™

At the American Heart Association, we want people to experience more of life's precious moments. That's why we've made better heart and brain health our mission. It's also why we remain committed to exceptional training—the act of bringing resuscitation science to life—through genuine partnership with you. Only through our continued collaboration and dedication can we truly make a difference and save lives.

Until there's a world free of heart disease and stroke, the American Heart Association will be there, working with you to make a healthier, longer life possible for everyone.

Why do we do what we do?
life is why.

Life Is Why is a celebration of life. A simple yet powerful answer to the question of why we should all be healthy in heart and mind. It also explains why we do what we do: Lifesaving work. Every day.

Throughout your student manual, you will find information that correlates what you are learning in this class to **Life Is Why** and the importance of cardiovascular care. Look for the **Life Is Why** icon (shown at right), and remember that what you are learning today has an impact on the mission of the American Heart Association.

We encourage you to discover your **Why** and share it with others. Ask yourself, what are the moments, people, and experiences I live for? What brings me joy, wonder, and happiness? Why am I partnering with the AHA to help save lives? Why is cardiovascular care important to me? The answer to these questions is your **Why.**

Instructions

Please find on the back of this page a chance for you to participate in the AHA's mission and **Life Is Why** campaign. Complete this activity by filling in the blank with the word that describes your **Why.**

Share your "_____ Is Why" with the people you love, and ask them to discover their **Why.**

Talk about it. Share it. Post it. Live it.   **#lifeiswhy**   **#CPRSavesLives**

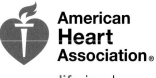

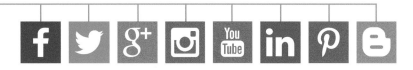

is why.

American Heart Association®

life is why™

Introduction

Heartsaver Pediatric First Aid CPR AED Course

Welcome to the Heartsaver® Pediatric First Aid CPR AED Course. During this course, you will gain knowledge and skills that may help save a life.

In this course, you will learn the basics of pediatric first aid, the most common life-threatening emergencies, how to recognize them, and how to help. You will also learn how to recognize when someone needs CPR, how to call for help, and how to give CPR and use an AED.

What You Will Learn in This Course

In this course, you will learn the key steps of pediatric first aid and how to provide care for a wide range of first aid emergencies. You will learn how to respond to first aid emergencies that are not life threatening. However, if a serious emergency does occur, you will be prepared to respond.

An important goal of this course is to teach you to act in emergency situations. Sometimes, people don't act because they are afraid of doing the wrong thing. Recognizing that something is wrong and getting help on the way by phoning 9-1-1 are the most important things you can do.

Life Is Why

Life Is Why

At the American Heart Association, we want people to experience more of life's precious moments. What you learn in this course can help build healthier, longer lives for everyone.

Heartsaver Pediatric First Aid CPR AED Knowledge and Skills

To respond to a first aid emergency, you will need both knowledge and skills:

- Knowledge is what you need to know, such as what to do if a child has swallowed a poison.
- Skills are what you need to do, such as controlling bleeding by direct pressure and bandaging or performing high-quality CPR.

Your Student Workbook contains all of the information that you need to be able to understand and perform lifesaving and first aid skills correctly. During the course, you will have the opportunity to practice certain skills and get valuable coaching from your instructor.

The video in the course will cover many, but not all, of the skills discussed in this workbook. So it is important to study your workbook to be fully prepared to help in an emergency.

Successful Course Completion

During the course, you will have an opportunity to practice and demonstrate important skills. As you read and study this workbook, pay particular attention to these skills.

If you complete all course requirements and demonstrate the skills correctly, you'll receive a course completion card.

How to Use the Student Workbook

Take time to read and study the Student Workbook carefully. You should use this workbook before, during, and after the course.

Before the course	• Read and study the workbook. • Look at the step-by-step instructions, skills summaries, and pictures. • Take notes. • Review your employer's policies and procedures that apply to first aid. For example, if you work in a childcare center, review what you should do in a first aid emergency. Know how to get help, whom to contact, and steps for follow-up. • Make a list of questions to ask your instructor.
During the course	• Refer to the workbook during the video demonstrations and hands-on practice.
After the course	• Review the step-by-step instructions, skills summaries, and pictures. • Keep your workbook readily available for reference during emergencies.

How Often Training Is Needed

Review your Student Workbook and Quick Reference Guide often to recall important skills. Your course completion card is valid for 2 years.

Pediatric First Aid Course Objectives

This course includes both first aid and CPR AED. At the end of the First Aid portion, you will be able to do the following to help in a first aid emergency:

- List the priorities, roles, and responsibilities of a rescuer providing first aid to a child or infant
- Describe the 4 key steps in first aid for children and infants: prevent, protect, assess, and act
- Remove protective gloves (skill you will demonstrate)
- Find the problem (skill you will demonstrate)

- Describe the assessment and first aid actions for the following life-threatening conditions: difficulty breathing, choking, severe bleeding, and shock
- Control bleeding and bandaging (skill you will demonstrate)
- Use an epinephrine pen (skill you will demonstrate)
- Recognize elements of common injuries
- Recognize elements of common illnesses
- Describe how to find information on preventing illness and injury
- Recognize the legal questions that apply to pediatric first aid rescuers

Heartsaver Pediatric First Aid CPR AED Terms and Concepts

What You Will Learn

In this section, you'll learn key terms and concepts that are used throughout this Heartsaver Course. They are the foundation for understanding the material presented in this workbook.

First Aid

First aid is the immediate care that you give a child with an illness or injury. This care may help an ill or injured child recover more completely or more quickly. In serious emergencies, first aid can mean the difference between life and death.

First aid may be started by anyone in any situation. Most of the time, you'll give first aid for minor illnesses or injuries. But you may also give first aid for problems that could become life threatening. This includes applying pressure to stop severe bleeding or giving epinephrine for a severe allergic reaction.

In this course, you will learn and practice first aid skills. This will help you remember what to do in a real emergency.

Responsive vs Unresponsive

You should know that during an emergency, it's possible that a child might become unresponsive. Here is how to decide if a child is responsive or unresponsive:

- *Responsive:* A child who is responsive will move, speak, blink, or otherwise react to you when you tap him and ask if he's OK.
- *Unresponsive:* A child who does not move, speak, blink, or otherwise react is unresponsive.

If a child is unresponsive, you will learn to check to see if the child needs CPR.

Agonal Gasps

A child in cardiac arrest will not be breathing or only gasping. When we refer to *gasps*, we mean agonal gasps. Agonal gasps are often present in the first minutes after sudden cardiac arrest.

If a child is gasping, it usually looks like he is drawing air in very quickly. He may open his mouth and move his jaw, head, or neck.

The gasp may sound like a snort, snore, or groan. These gasps may appear forceful or weak. Some time may pass between gasps because they often happen at a slow rate.

Gasping is not regular or normal breathing. It's a sign of cardiac arrest in a child who is unresponsive.

Cardiopulmonary Resuscitation

CPR stands for cardiopulmonary resuscitation. When a child's heart stops suddenly, providing CPR can double or even triple the chance of survival.

CPR is made up of 2 skills:

- Providing compressions
- Giving breaths

A *compression* is the act of pushing hard and fast on the chest. When you push on the chest, you pump blood to the brain and heart. To give CPR, you provide sets of 30 compressions and 2 breaths.

See the "CPR and AED" part of this workbook for more information.

Automated External Defibrillator

AED stands for automated external defibrillator. It's a lightweight, portable device that can detect an abnormal cardiac rhythm that needs to be treated with a shock. An AED can deliver a shock to stop abnormal electrical activity that often causes cardiac arrest. This allows the heart's normal rhythm to resume.

When you give first aid, you will need to get the first aid kit and sometimes an AED. AEDs should be located in a company's main office, a building's high-traffic area, a break room, or a high-risk area, such as a gym—any place where most people can see and get to them in an emergency.

It is very important that you become aware of the location of the nearest first aid kit and AED. Then you will be able to provide the best possible first aid care to someone who is ill or injured.

Adults, Children, and Infants

This workbook presents specific Heartsaver skills and actions for helping an ill or injured child or infant until the next level of care arrives. For the purposes of this course, we use the following age definitions:

Adult	Adolescent (after the onset of puberty) and older
Child	1 year old to puberty
Infant	Less than 1 year old

Signs of puberty include chest or underarm hair in males and any breast development in females.

Treat anyone who has signs of puberty as an adult. If you are in doubt about whether someone is an adult or a child, provide emergency care as if the child is an adult.

Phone 9-1-1

In this course, we say "phone 9-1-1." You may have a different emergency response number. If you do, phone your emergency response number instead of 9-1-1.

In an emergency, use the most readily available phone to phone 9-1-1. This may be your cell phone or the cell phone of someone who comes to help. In some cases, you may need to use another type of phone. After phoning 9-1-1, make sure the phone is on speaker mode, if possible. This will allow the person providing emergency care to talk to the dispatcher.

Part 1: First Aid Basics

Topics Covered

Topics covered in this part are

- Duties, roles, and responsibilities of the first aid rescuer
- Key steps of first aid

As you read and study this part, pay particular attention to these 2 skills that you will be asked to demonstrate during the course:

Skills	• Removing protective gloves
	• Finding the problem

Duties, Roles, and Responsibilities of the First Aid Rescuer

Your Role

Your Role as a First Aid Rescuer

First aid is the immediate care that you give to a child with an illness or injury. Your role as a first aid rescuer is to

- Recognize that an emergency exists
- Make sure the scene is safe for you and the ill or injured child
- Phone or send someone to phone 9-1-1
- Provide care until someone with more advanced training arrives and takes over

Emergency Medical Services

When you phone 9-1-1, you activate the network of emergency providers—also called *emergency medical services* (EMS). Getting help on the way quickly in an emergency can save a life.

Your Duty to Maintain the First Aid Kit

The first aid kit should contain the supplies you'll need in the most common emergencies. One of the responsibilities of a first aid provider is to maintain the first aid kit.

Determine what you should keep in your kit. See the "Sample First Aid Kit" in "Part 5: First Aid Resources" for suggestions. You may need different supplies depending on the type of facility and geographic location.

It's important that the first aid kit contain the supplies you'll need for most common emergencies. Be sure to restock it after any emergency.

☐ Keep the supplies in a sturdy, watertight container that is clearly labeled.

☐ Know where the first aid kit is.

☐ Replace what you use so that the kit will be ready for the next emergency.

☐ Check the kit at the beginning of each work period for expired supplies. Make sure it is complete and ready for an emergency.

Plans for First Aid Emergencies

Every childcare facility and school should be prepared for an illness or injury emergency. A plan for such emergencies includes the

- Emergency response number (usually 9-1-1)
- Location of the first aid kit and AED
- Location of where medicines are stored
- Other information, such as
  - Names of people in the facility who have first aid training
  - Telephone numbers and locations of nearby emergency care facilities
  - Telephone number of the poison control center (1-800-222-1222)

First Aid Action Plans

Schools and childcare facilities should have a health record and written first aid action plan for each child with a medical condition. The first aid action plan describes what to do for a related medical emergency. For example, the plan gives instructions for what to do if the child has an asthma attack, a severe allergic reaction, or a seizure.

A first aid action plan usually includes

- Medical history and medicines
- How and when to give the medicines
- Other actions to take if the child becomes ill
- Contact information for parents or caregivers
- Name and telephone number of the child's healthcare provider

See an example of a first aid action plan in "Part 5: First Aid Resources."

Special Medical Devices

Some children with special needs may use certain medical devices. A child with diabetes, for example, may have an insulin pump. If you have a child with special needs in your care, learn about what devices the child uses, if any.

Plan for Storing and Managing Medicines	Make sure you know where your facility stores medicines. They should be stored in a way that - Protects the privacy of the child - Keeps them out of children's reach Other plans may be needed for storage and management, such as checking expiration dates.
Emergency Response Plan	All schools, childcare facilities, and even families should have an emergency response plan. It's important to be prepared to respond quickly and efficiently in an emergency.

Your Responsibilities

Barriers and Benefits	Sometimes rescuers worry about doing the right thing to help in an emergency. Sometimes rescuers are overwhelmed by the sight of an injury. By taking this course and learning first aid skills, you will increase your confidence and ability to respond in emergency situations. This will improve your ability to help when a child or infant becomes ill or injured.
Confidentiality	As a first aid rescuer, you will learn private things about children's medical conditions. Give information about an ill or injured child only to caregivers, a healthcare provider, and anyone with more training who takes over from you. You may also need to fill out a report if your employer or company requires it. Don't share this information, except as required. Keep private things private.
Good Samaritan Laws	If you have questions about whether or not it's legal to provide first aid, you should know that all states have Good Samaritan laws. These laws protect anyone who provides first aid. They differ from state to state, so be sure to check the laws in your area.

The key steps of pediatric first aid will guide you in caring for an ill or injured child.

4 Key Steps of Pediatric First Aid

For every pediatric first aid emergency, follow these steps:

1	**Prevent**	Keep children from getting hurt.
2	**Protect**	Keep yourself and the ill or injured child safe.
3	**Assess**	Recognize the problem and know when to phone 9-1-1.
4	**Act**	Give first aid and phone 9-1-1 if needed.

Step 1: Prevent

One of the best ways to prevent injury is to watch children and take steps to prevent an injury from happening. For example, if you see a child reach for a hot pan, you can stop her before she gets burned.

Many injuries can be prevented by performing simple actions in the home, car, childcare center, school, and playground. See "Part 4: Preventing Illness and Injury" for more information on how to keep children safe.

Step 2: Protect

Most first aid rescuers know how important it is to protect an ill or injured child. It's also important to protect yourself. You can't help anyone if you are ill or injured yourself. Do the following before giving first aid care:

- Make sure the scene is safe for you and the child.
- Wash your hands to protect yourself and others from disease.
- Wear protective gloves. Remove the gloves properly. This will keep you from being exposed to blood or bodily fluids.
- Wear other protective equipment as needed. This may include masks and eye protection.

Assess the Scene

Assess the scene to make sure it is safe. Be aware of any danger for you, the ill or injured child, and anyone else nearby. Sometimes your efforts to help can put you in danger. For example, if a child is injured in a car crash in heavy traffic, you should watch for other cars.

Make sure the scene is safe. This is an important step. Do it every time you are providing help. Continue to assess the scene while you give first aid. You need to be aware of anything that might change and make it unsafe. You can't help if you're injured yourself.

Questions for Assessing the Scene

When you look around, ask yourself these questions:

	Question	Explanation
Danger	Is there danger for you or the ill or injured child?	Move an injured child only if he is in danger or if you need to move him to safely provide first aid or CPR.
Help	Are others around to help?	If so, send someone to phone 9-1-1. If no one else is near, phone for help yourself.
Who	Who is ill or injured?	Can you tell how many people are hurt and what happened?
Where	Where are you?	You'll need to tell others how to get to you—in particular, the 9-1-1 dispatcher. If there are other bystanders at the scene, send one of them to meet the emergency providers and lead them to the scene.

Phone for Help

Phoning for help and getting EMS providers on the way quickly can be the most important thing to do in an emergency.

Always be aware of your location. This will help emergency providers reach you more quickly.

Make sure you know the nearest location of a phone to use in an emergency (Figure 1). Often, the first aid kit and AED are stored at the same location as the emergency phone.

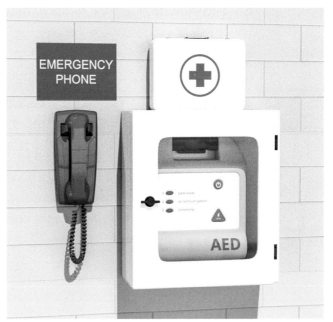

Figure 1. Know the location of the nearest phone to use in an emergency. You also should know where the first aid kit and AED are stored.

When to Phone for Help

Your facility's emergency action plan or the child's First Aid Action Plan may have instructions about when to phone 9-1-1. As a general rule, you should phone 9-1-1 for the following emergencies:

Phone 9-1-1 and Ask for Help If
☐ The child is seriously ill or injured
☐ You are not sure what to do in an emergency

Some examples of when you should phone 9-1-1 are if the ill or injured child

- Doesn't respond to voice or touch
- Has severe bleeding
- Has a severe allergic reaction
- Has a problem breathing
- Has a severe injury or burn
- Has received an electric shock
- Suddenly can't move a part of the body
- Has swallowed or been exposed to poison
- Has a seizure
- Has tried to commit suicide
- Has been assaulted

You will learn more about the signs and first aid actions for medical and injury emergencies later in this workbook.

How to Phone for Help

It's also important for you to know how to phone for help from your location. Do you know how to activate the emergency response number in your workplace? For example, do you need to dial 9 for an outside line? Is there an internal number to phone that will notify emergency providers who are on-site?

For the purposes of this course, we will say "phone 9-1-1" as the emergency response number.

Write the emergency response number on your Quick Reference Guide, in the first aid kit, and near the telephone. You should also write it here.

Write your emergency response number here:

_____

Who Should Phone for Help

If other people are available, you can send someone else to phone 9-1-1 and get the first aid kit and AED. If you are alone and have a cell phone, phone 9-1-1. Put the phone on speaker mode so that you can follow the dispatcher's instructions. Here is a summary:

If you are	Then you should
Alone	☐ Shout for help. ☐ If no one answers and the child needs immediate care and you have a cell phone, phone 9-1-1. Put the phone on speaker mode. ☐ The dispatcher will provide further instruction. She may tell you how to give first aid, give CPR, or use an AED.
With others	☐ Stay with the ill or injured child. Be prepared to give first aid or CPR if you know how. ☐ Send someone else to phone 9-1-1 and get the first aid kit and AED if available. ☐ Ask the person to put the phone on speaker mode so that you can hear instructions from the dispatcher.

When to Notify Parents and Caregivers

It's important to phone 9-1-1 before phoning anyone else. Notify parents and caregivers about any first aid the child received as soon as you have finished caring for the child or after advanced care arrives and takes over.

Follow the Dispatcher's Instructions

When you're on the phone with the dispatcher, don't hang up until the dispatcher tells you to. Answering the dispatcher's questions won't delay arrival of help.

Take Universal Precautions

Before you assess the child, you should take universal precautions. These precautions are called *universal* because you should treat all blood and other body fluids as if they contain germs that can cause diseases. Other body fluids include saliva and urine.

Personal Protective Equipment

Your first aid kit includes personal protective equipment (or PPE). Some types of PPE are eye protection and medical gloves. While you are giving first aid, these help keep you safe from blood and body fluids. The first aid kit also may contain a mask for giving breaths during CPR.

You should use nonlatex gloves if possible. Some people are allergic to latex. Others have a sensitivity to latex that can result in serious allergic reactions.

Universal Precautions

Take the following actions to protect yourself from disease and injury:

Universal Precautions

☐ Wear PPE whenever necessary (Figure 2).
  • Wear protective gloves whenever you give first aid.
  • Wear eye protection if the ill or injured child is bleeding.

☐ Place all disposable equipment that has touched blood or touched body fluids containing blood in a biohazard waste bag (Figure 3) or as required by your workplace.

☐ To dispose of the biohazard waste bag, follow your company's plan for disposing of hazardous waste.

☐ After properly removing your gloves, wash your hands well with soap and lots of water for 20 seconds.

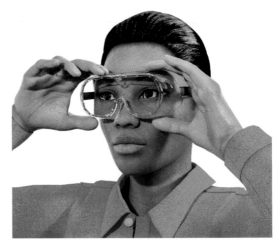

Figure 2. Wear protective gloves whenever you give first aid. Wear eye protection if the ill or injured child is bleeding.

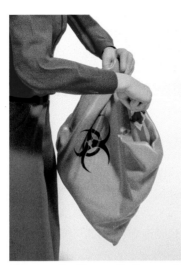
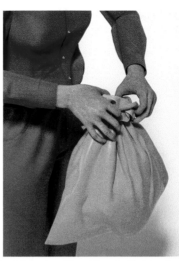

Figure 3. Place all disposable equipment that has touched body fluids, including the gloves you wore, in a biohazard waste bag if one is available. Dispose of the bag according to company policy.

Exposure to Blood or Other Body Fluids

You should always wear PPE whenever possible. However, if the child's blood or other body fluids do make contact with your skin, or splash in your eyes or mouth, take these steps:

What to Do If Exposed to Blood or Other Body Fluids
☐ Remove your gloves if you are wearing them.
☐ Immediately wash your hands. Rinse the contact area with soap and lots of water for 20 seconds.
☐ If body fluids splattered in your eyes, your nose, or the inside of your mouth, rinse the area with plenty of water.
☐ Contact a healthcare provider as soon as possible.

Remove Protective Gloves

Because of the risk of infection, it is important to use protective gloves and take them off correctly. This will help keep you and others safe.

Always dispose of protective gloves properly. This protects others who come in contact with the biohazard waste bag from being exposed to blood or body fluids.

How to Remove Protective Gloves

Here is the correct way to remove protective gloves (Figure 4):

How to Remove Protective Gloves

☐ Grip one glove on the outside near the cuff. Peel it down until it comes off inside out (Figure 4A).

☐ Cup it with your other gloved hand (Figure 4B).

☐ Place 2 fingers of your bare hand inside the cuff of the glove that is still on your other hand (Figure 4C).

☐ Peel that glove off so that it comes off inside out with the first glove inside it (Figure 4D).

☐ If blood or blood-containing material is on the gloves, dispose of the gloves properly.
  • Put the gloves in a biohazard waste bag.
  • If you do not have a biohazard waste bag, put the gloves in a plastic bag that can be sealed before you dispose of it.

☐ Wash your hands well. You should always wash your hands after removing gloves, just in case some blood or body fluids came in contact with your hands.

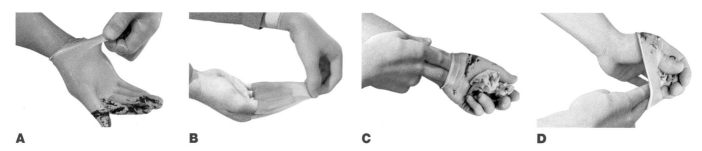

A   B   C   D

Figure 4. Proper removal of protective gloves without touching the outside of the gloves.

Practice Good Hand Hygiene

Even if you've been wearing protective gloves, you should always wash your hands. This is in case some blood or body fluids came in contact with your hands. Also, good hand hygiene helps prevent the spread of germs. Washing your hands well is important protection against infection.

How to Wash Hands Well

☐ Wet your hands with clean running water (warm if available) and apply soap.

☐ Rub hands together; scrub all surfaces of hands and fingers for at least 20 seconds (Figure 5).

☐ Rinse hands with lots of running water.

☐ Dry your hands using a paper towel or air dryer. If possible, use your paper towel to turn off the faucet.

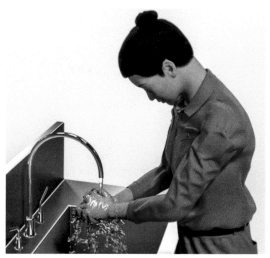

Figure 5. After taking off your gloves, wash your hands well with soap and lots of water for at least 20 seconds.

Using Waterless Hand Sanitizer

If you can't wash your hands right away, use waterless hand sanitizer. Rub your hands together so that the sanitizer covers the tops and bottoms of both hands and all fingers. Let the sanitizer air dry.

Then as soon as you can, wash your hands with soap and water.

How Children Act When Something Is Wrong

To find out if something is wrong with a child, notice how the child is acting. Interact with the child in a calm and comforting way. Then, follow the steps for finding the problem.

How Children Act When Something Is Wrong

Sometimes you can't tell right away if a child is ill or injured. All you may notice is that the child is not acting like himself—that is, he is not acting the same way he usually acts. This may mean that he is ill or injured.

Ill or injured children may act younger than they are. Respond to them based on their behavior, not their age.

To learn more about what kinds of behavior to expect from children of different ages, see "How Children Act and Tips for Interacting With Them" in Part 5.

Interacting With an Ill or Injured Child

Calm and comfort an ill or injured child. Here are some tips:

Tips for Calming and Comforting an Ill or Injured Child	
Be calm, direct, and clear	☐ If you are calm, you have the best chance to talk to and help a child. • Even infants will respond to your calm tone of voice, if not your actual words. • Toddlers who can usually speak well may not be able to do so in emergencies. They may bite or act angry when frustrated. • Adolescents may not want to talk. ☐ Don't disregard a child's complaints and concerns, no matter how old the child is. Make it clear that you are listening carefully.
Get down to the child's level	Kneel, squat, or sit to get down to the child's level when you talk to him. This often helps reduce the child's fear.
Move gently	If a child is afraid, gentle motions may calm her.

Know When to Phone 9-1-1

Recognize when the child's illness or injury is serious or life threatening. The child may need more help than you can provide. Knowing when to phone 9-1-1 is very important in providing first aid.

Find the Problem

Before you give first aid, you must find out what the problem is.

- Check to see if the child is responsive or unresponsive. If the child is unresponsive, check for breathing.
- If the child is breathing and doesn't need immediate first aid, look for any obvious signs of injury, such as bleeding, broken bones, burns, or bites.
- Look for any medical information jewelry (Figure 6). This tells you if the child has a serious medical condition.
- Follow the actions outlined in "Steps for Finding the Problem."

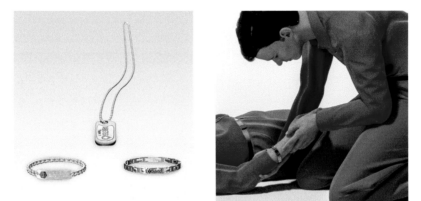

Figure 6. Look for medical information jewelry.

Steps for Finding the Problem

The following steps will help you find out what the problem is. They are listed in order of importance, with the most important step listed first.

Steps for Finding the Problem
☐ Make sure the scene is safe.

☐ Check to see if the child responds (Figure 7). Approach the child, tap him, and shout, "Are you OK? Are you OK?"

If the child is *responsive*	If the child is *unresponsive*
☐ Ask what the problem is if the child is old enough to talk.	☐ Shout for help and send someone to phone 9-1-1 and get a first aid kit and AED (Figure 8).
☐ If the child only moves, moans, or groans, shout for help. Phone or send someone to phone 9-1-1 and get the first aid kit and AED.	☐ Stay with the child. • If you are alone and no one comes to help and you have a cell phone, phone 9-1-1. Put the phone on speaker mode.

(continued)

(continued)

If the child is *responsive*	If the child is *unresponsive*

☐ Check the child's breathing.
  • If the child is breathing without difficulty and doesn't need immediate first aid, continue finding the problem.
  • If the child is having breathing problems, help him. See "Breathing Problems (Asthma)" in Part 2.
	☐ Check for breathing (Figure 9).
	  • If the child is breathing, roll him onto his side (if you don't think he has a neck or back injury). Phone 9-1-1 if no one has already done so. Stay with the child until advanced help arrives.
	  • If the child is not breathing or is only gasping, perform 2 minutes of CPR. Then, if no one has done so, phone 9-1-1 and get an AED. See the "CPR and AED" part of this workbook.

☐ Check for any obvious signs of injury, such as bleeding, broken bones, burns, or bites.	☐ Check for any obvious signs of injury, such as bleeding, broken bones, burns, or bites.
☐ Look for any medical information jewelry. This will tell you if the child has a serious medical condition.	☐ Look for any medical information jewelry. This will tell you if the child has a serious medical condition.
☐ If the child is seriously ill or injured or you don't know what to do, phone 9-1-1. Stay with the child until someone with more advanced training arrives and takes over.	☐ Stay with the child until someone with more advanced training arrives and takes over.

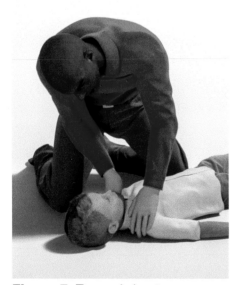

Figure 7. Tap and shout.

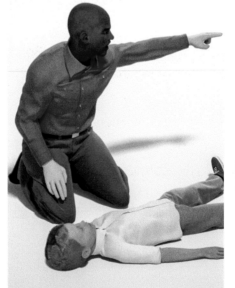

Figure 8. Get help.

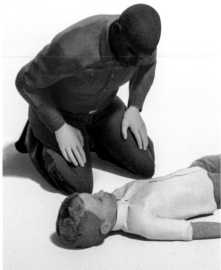

Figure 9. Check breathing.

Check the Child Often

A child's condition can change quickly. A child may respond and then stop responding, so check the child often.

When a child does not respond, he may stop breathing. Watch carefully to make sure that the child keeps breathing. If the child doesn't respond and is not breathing, give CPR.

Use Caution When Moving an Ill or Injured Child

When giving first aid, you might wonder, "Should I move an ill or injured child?"

The answer is generally no. It is especially important to avoid moving a child if you suspect a head, back, spinal, or pelvic injury.

However, there are times when the child should be moved, such as the following:

- If the area is unsafe for you or the ill or injured child, move to a safe location.
- If a child is unresponsive and breathing (and you don't suspect head, neck, spinal, or pelvic injury), you may roll the child onto his side. Rolling the child onto his side may help keep his airway open in case he vomits.

One way to move the child is to drag him by his clothes. Place your hands on the child's shoulders, grab his clothes, and pull him to safety.

What to Do If You Suspect Child Abuse

In many states, anyone who suspects child abuse is required to report it. By reporting what you learned, you may help protect the child from future injury and even death. See "Child Abuse and Neglect" in Part 5.

Step 4: Act

After you have assessed the child and found the problem, the next step is to *act* to provide first aid care.

We want you to act in an emergency. Sometimes, people don't act because they are afraid of doing the wrong thing. Knowing when to phone 9-1-1 is a critical part of first aid care. Two of the most important things you can do are

- Recognize that something is wrong
- Get help on the way

Dispatchers—the people who answer 9-1-1 calls—can tell you what to do in serious emergencies. People with more training (emergency medical technicians, paramedics, and others) usually arrive and take over not long after you call.

2 Groups of Illnesses and Injuries

The illnesses and injuries covered in this workbook are divided into 2 groups:

Group A	Illnesses and injuries that can become serious very quickly unless the child gets first aid care right away
Group B	Illnesses and injuries that may not be as urgent but still can become serious without first aid care and follow-up

First Aid Basics: Review Questions

Question	Your Notes
1. What is the most important thing that you can do in an emergency? a. Don't do anything unless you are sure what to do b. Hope someone else comes who is better prepared c. Phone 9-1-1 d. Pretend you don't see the ill or injured child	
2. Duties as a first aid rescuer include a. Maintaining the first aid kit b. Keeping private information about the ill or injured child private c. Understanding laws in your state that protect anyone who provides first aid d. All of the above	
3. What is the most important step in preventing illness? a. Posting the poison control number near a phone b. Wearing a mask c. Putting all blood-containing material into a leak-proof bag d. Handwashing	

(continued)

Question	Your Notes
4. The purpose of taking your gloves off properly is to keep blood or fluids on the gloves from touching your skin. True False	
5. Why is it important to answer all of the dispatcher's questions? a. Because the 9-1-1 dispatcher needs to complete a survey b. Because it will get help to you as fast as possible c. To keep yourself safe so that you don't become injured too d. So the dispatcher can give a report to the media	
6. When giving first aid to a child or infant, when should you phone 9-1-1? a. For every first aid emergency b. For a serious illness or injury c. If the child or infant has a fever and does not have a First Aid Action Plan d. Anytime bleeding is present	
7. Which of the following may be true about how a child acts when something is wrong? a. The child may act ill or injured. b. The child may act younger than she is. c. The child may need for you to talk to her based on her behavior, not her age. d. All of the above	

(continued)

Question	Your Notes
8. If you are not sure what is wrong with a child, you'll need to find the problem. What is the first step you should take? a. Check for injuries or medical jewelry b. Check for breathing c. Make sure the scene is safe d. Check for a response (tap and shout)	

Answers: 1. c, 2. d, 3. d, 4. True, 5. b, 6. b, 7. d, 8. c

Part 2: Illnesses and Injuries: Group A

Group A includes illnesses and injuries you may encounter that can become serious very quickly. You'll need to act fast in these situations. Your first aid actions can make an immediate difference.

Topics Covered

Topics covered in this part are

- External bleeding
- Internal bleeding
- Burns
- Allergic reactions
- Breathing problems (asthma)
- Dehydration
- Diabetes and low blood sugar
- Heat-related emergencies
- Cold-related emergencies
- Drowning

As you read and study this part, pay particular attention to these 2 skills that you will be asked to demonstrate during the course:

| Skills | • Control bleeding by direct pressure and bandaging |
| | • Use an epinephrine pen |

External Bleeding

Bleeding can be either external or internal. External bleeding is bleeding outside the skin that you can see. Internal bleeding is bleeding inside the skin that you can't see. This section covers what to do for external bleeding. External bleeding can quickly become life threatening if not controlled.

Severe bleeding occurs when a large blood vessel is cut or torn. When this happens, a child can lose a lot of blood within minutes. Severe bleeding may be stopped with pressure applied over the cut or tear.

Minor bleeding occurs from small cuts or scrapes. Most bleeding can be stopped with pressure. You'll use less direct pressure to stop the bleeding for a minor cut or scrape than for a major cut or scrape.

It's important to stay calm. Bleeding often looks worse than it is.

Dressing vs Bandage

Many people confuse the terms *dressing* and *bandage*. Here is what they mean and how they work together:

- A *dressing* is a clean material used directly on a wound to stop bleeding. It can be a piece of gauze or any other clean piece of cloth.
- A *bandage* is material used to protect or cover an injured body part. A bandage also may be used to help keep pressure on a wound.

If needed, you can hold gauze dressings in place over a wound with a bandage (Figure 10).

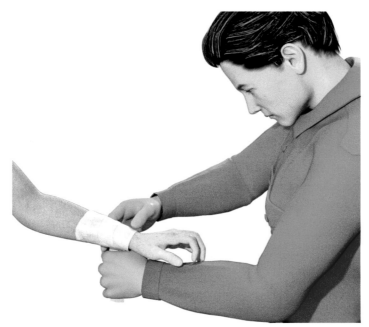

Figure 10. Placing a bandage over a dressing.

When to Phone 9-1-1 for Bleeding

Phone or send someone to phone 9-1-1 if

- There is a lot of bleeding
- You cannot stop the bleeding
- You see signs of shock (see "Shock" later in this Part)
- You suspect a head, neck, or spinal injury
- You are not sure what to do

Step 1: Prevent
- Use the Child and Infant Safety Checklist to help keep a child safe.
- Use dressings to help prevent infection.
- Use antibiotic cream on small scrapes and surface cuts to prevent infection. (Make sure the child doesn't have an allergy to antibiotic cream first.)

Step 2: Protect
- Make sure the scene is safe.
- Get the first aid kit.
- Wear PPE.
- If the injured child can help you, ask him to put direct pressure on the wound while you put on your PPE.

Step 3: Assess
Find the place that's bleeding.

Control Bleeding by Direct Pressure and Bandaging

Step 4: Act
Follow these steps to stop bleeding:

How to Control Bleeding With Direct Pressure and Bandaging
☐ Apply dressings from the first aid kit. Put direct pressure on the dressings over the bleeding area. Use the flat part of your fingers or the palm of your hand (Figure 11).
☐ If the bleeding doesn't stop, you'll need to add more dressings and press harder. Do not remove a dressing once it's in place because this could cause the wound to bleed more. Keep pressure on the wound until it stops bleeding.
☐ Once the bleeding has stopped or if you can't keep pressure on the wound, wrap a bandage firmly over the dressings to hold them in place.
☐ For minor cuts and scrapes, wash the area with soap and water once the bleeding has stopped. Then apply a dressing to the wound.

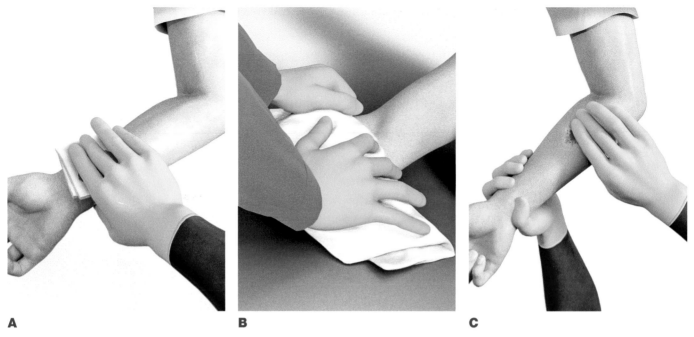

A **B** **C**

Figure 11. Controlling bleeding. **A**, A dressing can be a gauze pad or pads. **B**, It can be any other clean piece of cloth. **C**, If you do not have a dressing, use your gloved hand.

Use a Tourniquet

If an arm or leg has severe bleeding and you can't stop the bleeding with direct pressure, you can use a tourniquet. Be sure you phone 9-1-1 and get an AED, if available. Uncontrolled bleeding can lead to more complications.

The first aid kit may contain a premade or manufactured tourniquet. It includes a strap that you wrap around the injured child's arm or leg and a straight, stick-like object called a *windlass*. The windlass is used to tighten the tourniquet. If applied correctly, a tourniquet should stop the bleeding.

If you apply the tourniquet correctly, it will cause pain as it stops the bleeding.

Once you have the tourniquet in place, note the time. Leave it alone until someone with more advanced training arrives and takes over.

How to Apply a Premade Tourniquet

Follow these steps to apply a premade tourniquet from your first aid kit:

How to Apply a Premade Tourniquet
☐ Make sure the scene is safe.
☐ Phone or send someone to phone 9-1-1 and get the first aid kit (if you do not already have it) and an AED.
☐ Wear PPE.
☐ Place the tourniquet about 2 inches above the injury if possible.
☐ Tighten the tourniquet until the bleeding stops.
☐ Note what time the tourniquet was placed on the body.
☐ Once you have the tourniquet in place and the bleeding has stopped, leave it alone until someone with more advanced training arrives and takes over.

How to Make and Apply a Tourniquet

If you don't have a tourniquet, you can make one. Follow these steps to make and apply a tourniquet:

How to Make and Apply a Tourniquet
☐ Make sure the scene is safe.
☐ Phone or send someone to phone 9-1-1 and get the first aid kit (if you do not already have it) and an AED.
☐ Wear PPE.
☐ Fold a cloth or bandage so that it's long and at least 1 inch wide.
☐ Wrap the bandage 2 inches above the injury if possible.
☐ Tie the ends of the bandage around a small hand tool, stick, or something similar.
☐ Turn the hand tool or stick (or other object) to tighten the tourniquet.
☐ Continue tightening until the bleeding stops.
☐ Secure the hand tool or stick so the tourniquet stays tight.
☐ Note what time the tourniquet was placed.
☐ Once you have the tourniquet in place and the bleeding has stopped, leave it alone until someone with more advanced training arrives and takes over.

Shock can be caused by losing a large amount of blood or water. It develops when not enough blood flows to the most important parts of the body. It is not an illness a child can just "get." Another illness or injury always causes it. Shock can be fatal.

Watch for shock, especially if a child is not acting like himself and he

- Has recently lost a lot of fluid, such as with vomiting or diarrhea
- Has a fever and has not taken in enough fluid
- Loses a lot of blood, including bleeding inside the body
- Has a severe allergic reaction

Step 1: Prevent

Use the Child and Infant Safety Checklist to help prevent injuries that lead to severe bleeding.

Step 2: Protect

- Make sure the scene is safe.
- Get the first aid kit and AED.
- Wear PPE.

Step 3: Assess

A child in shock doesn't act like herself. Signs of shock include

- Feeling weak, faint, or dizzy
- Being nauseated
- Breathing very fast
- Acting restless, confused, or unusually sleepy
- Looking pale
- Being cold to the touch

Step 4: Act

Follow these steps to help a child in shock (Figure 12):

How to Help a Child Who Is in Shock
☐ Phone or send someone to phone 9-1-1 and get the first aid kit and AED.
☐ Help the child lie on his back.
☐ Cover the child with a blanket to keep him warm.
☐ Remain with the child until someone with advanced training arrives and takes over.
☐ Give CPR if the child doesn't respond and is not breathing.

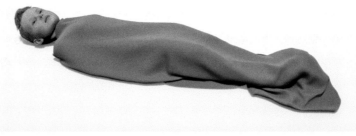

Figure 12. Cover a child who is in shock.

Internal Bleeding

Internal bleeding is bleeding inside the body. The skin may not be broken, so you may not be able to see blood or signs of bleeding. But something (an organ, a blood vessel) beneath the skin is cut, bruised, or torn and is bleeding inside the body. This kind of blood loss is serious. It can lead to shock.

When to Suspect Internal Bleeding

You should suspect internal bleeding if a child has

- An injury from a car crash
- Been hit by a car
- Fallen from a height
- An injury in the abdomen or chest (including bruises, such as seat belt marks)
- Sports injuries, such as slamming into other players or being hit with a ball
- Pain in the abdomen or chest after an injury
- Shortness of breath after an injury
- Coughed up or vomited blood after an injury
- Signs of shock without external bleeding
- A knife or a gunshot wound

Step 1: Prevent

Use the Child and Infant Safety Checklist to help prevent injuries that may lead to internal bleeding.

Step 2: Protect

- Make sure the scene is safe.
- Phone or send someone to phone 9-1-1 and get the first aid kit and AED.
- Wear PPE.

Step 3: Assess

A child with internal bleeding may develop shock. Signs of shock include

- Feeling weak, faint, or dizzy
- Being nauseated
- Breathing very fast
- Acting restless, confused, or unusually sleepy
- Looking pale
- Being cold to the touch

Step 4: Act

If you suspect internal bleeding, follow these steps:

How to Help a Child With Suspected Internal Bleeding
☐ Have the child lie down and keep still.
☐ Check for signs of shock.
☐ Phone or send someone to phone 9-1-1.
☐ Give CPR if the child doesn't respond and is not breathing.

Burns and Electrical Injuries

Burns

Burns are injuries that can be caused by contact with heat, electricity, or chemicals. Heat burns are caused when anyone comes in contact with a hot surface, hot liquids, steam, or fire.

The only thing you should put on a burn is cool water and clean dressings—never use ice. Ice can damage a burned area.

If the child has a burn, keep the child warm. If a skin burn is large, a child may not be able to control body temperature effectively. If the child gets too cold, low body temperature (hypothermia) can develop.

Step 1: Prevent   Take steps to prevent heat burns, chemical burns, and sunburns.

Preventing Heat Burns

- Keep hot foods and drinks out of children's reach.
- Don't hold a child or infant when cooking or working with something very hot.
- Make sure food isn't too hot before feeding it to children, especially infants.
- Be careful with small heating appliances or tools that have hot surfaces, such as curling irons.
  - Keep the appliance out children's reach.
  - Keep the cords out of reach so that children can't pull the appliance down.
  - Unplug appliances and tools when not in use.
- Adjust the hot water heater so that the water is 120° Fahrenheit or cooler. This will prevent scalding a child in a short time.

Preventing Chemical Burns

- Keep chemicals, such as bleach and drain cleaner, out of children's reach.

Preventing Sunburn

- Keep infants younger than 6 months old out of direct sunlight.
- Try to keep children out of the sun between 10 AM and 4 PM.
- For children older than 6 months, use sunscreen made for children.
- Put sunscreen on children 30 minutes before they go outside.
- Choose a water-resistant or waterproof sunscreen with a sun protection factor (SPF) of at least 15. The product should block long-wave and short-wave ultraviolet rays. So look for protection from both ultraviolet A (UVA) and ultraviolet B (UVB) rays.
- Reapply waterproof sunscreen every 2 hours. This is especially important if children are playing in the water.

Step 2: Protect

- Make sure the scene is safe.
- Get the first aid kit.
- Wear PPE.

Step 3: Assess   Assess the burned area to see if the burn is small or large. If the child or his clothing is on fire, take immediate action to put the fire out. Have the child stop, drop, and roll. Then cover the child with a wet blanket until the fire is out.

Step 4: Act

Take first aid steps based on whether the burned area is small or large.

How to Help a Child With Small Burns

☐ Cool the burned area immediately with cold (but not ice-cold) water for at least 10 minutes (Figure 13).

☐ If you do not have cold water, use a cool or cold (but not freezing) clean compress.

☐ Run cold water on the burn until it doesn't hurt.

☐ You may cover the burn with a dry, nonstick sterile or clean dressing.

How to Help a Child With Large Burns

☐ If there is a fire, the burn area is large, or you're not sure what to do, phone or send someone to phone 9-1-1.

☐ If the child or his clothing is on fire, put the fire out. Have the child stop, drop, and roll. Then cover the child with a wet blanket.

☐ Once the fire is out, remove the wet blanket. Carefully remove jewelry and clothing that is not stuck to the skin.

☐ For large burns, cool the burn area immediately with cold (but not ice-cold) water for at least 10 minutes.

☐ After you cool the burns, cover them with dry, nonstick sterile or clean dressings.

☐ Cover the child with a dry blanket.

☐ Check for signs of shock.

☐ A child with a large burn should be seen by a healthcare provider as soon as possible.

☐ A healthcare provider can decide if more treatment is needed.

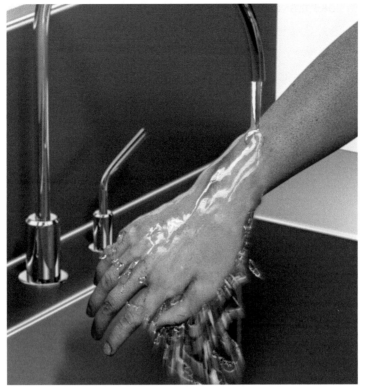

Figure 13. Cool burns immediately with cold (but not ice-cold) water.

Other First Aid for Burns

Many people have heard about different ointments for burns. The only thing you should put on a burn is cool water and clean dressings unless you are given other instructions by a healthcare provider.

Electrical Injuries

Electricity can cause burns on the outside of the body and on the inside, injuring organs. You may see marks or wounds where the electricity has entered and left the body. The damage can be severe. But there's no way to tell how severe based on the marks on the outside of the body. Electricity can stop a child from breathing. It can cause a deadly abnormal heart rhythm and cardiac arrest.

If an electrical injury is caused by high voltage, like a fallen power line, phone 9-1-1. Don't enter the area or try to move wires until the power has been turned off.

Step 1: Prevent

- Install "shock stops" (plastic outlet plugs) or outlet covers on all electrical outlets.
- Make sure cords are not frayed or cracked.
- Make sure plugs fit properly into the outlets.

Step 2: Protect

- Make sure the scene is safe.
- Get the first aid kit and AED.
- Wear PPE.
- Use caution before touching the child.
  - Don't touch the child if he is still in contact with the power source. Electricity can travel from the power source through the child to you. It's best to turn the power off, but only attempt this if you are trained to do so. Once the power is off, you may touch the injured child.
  - Don't touch anything that is in contact with a fallen power line or other high-voltage source. Electricity can travel through anything that comes in contact with a high-voltage source (even a wooden stick). Wait until the power has been turned off to enter the area. Then provide help.

Step 3: Assess

Look for burns and other injuries. Electricity may leave only small marks on the body. You can't tell how much damage there is inside the body based on the marks on the outside of the body.

Step 4: Act

Follow these steps to help a child with an electrical injury:

How to Help a Child With an Electrical Injury
☐ Use caution before touching the child (see Step 2: Protect).
☐ Phone or send someone to phone 9-1-1.
☐ When it is safe to touch the injured child, give CPR if the child doesn't respond and is not breathing or only gasping.
☐ A healthcare provider should check anyone who has an electrical injury as soon as possible.

Allergic Reactions

Allergies are quite common. A severe allergic reaction can quickly turn into a medical emergency.

Some things that can cause a severe allergic reaction are

- Eggs
- Peanuts
- Chocolate
- Some medicines
- Insect bites and stings, especially bee stings

Mild vs Severe Allergic Reaction

Here are some signs of mild and severe allergic reactions:

Signs of Mild Allergic Reaction	Signs of Severe Allergic Reaction
☐ A stuffy nose, sneezing, and itching around the eyes	☐ Trouble breathing
☐ Itching of the skin	☐ Swelling of the tongue and face
☐ Raised, red rash on the skin (hives)	☐ Signs of shock

Step 1: Prevent

Protect the child from things that are known to cause that child to develop an allergic reaction.

Step 2: Protect

- Make sure the scene is safe.
- Get the first aid kit.
- Wear PPE.

Step 3: Assess

Figure out whether the allergic reaction is mild or severe. Watch the child carefully. Some reactions that seem mild can become severe within minutes.

Step 4: Act

If the reaction is severe, phone or send someone to phone 9-1-1. You may need to use the child's epinephrine pen as directed by the child's First Aid Action Plan.

Epinephrine Pen for a Severe Allergic Reaction

Epinephrine is a drug that can stop a severe allergic reaction. The drug will help the child breathe more easily. In the United States, epinephrine is available by prescription in a self-injectable device. This device is sometimes called an *epinephrine pen*. People who are known to have severe allergic reactions are encouraged to carry epinephrine with them at all times.

Here are some points that you should know about the epinephrine pen:

- Some states and organizations permit first aid rescuers to help people use their epinephrine pens. People who carry epinephrine pens usually know when and how to use them.
- You may help give the injection if you are approved to do so by your state regulations.
- The epinephrine injection is given in the side of the thigh. It usually takes several minutes before the medicine starts to work.
- Epinephrine pens are not all alike. There are 2 doses of epinephrine pens—1 for adults and 1 for children.

■ Make sure you have the epinephrine pen that belongs to that child. If the child can't use the pen himself, and if you are allowed to, give him an injection.

Use an Epinephrine Pen

A severe allergic reaction can be life threatening. Follow these steps to help someone with signs of a severe allergic reaction use his epinephrine pen:

How to Use an Epinephrine Pen
☐ Follow the instructions on the pen. Make sure you are holding the pen in your fist without touching either end (because the needle comes out of one end). You may give the injection through clothes or on bare skin.
☐ Take off the safety cap (Figure 14A).
☐ Hold the leg firmly in place just before and during the injection. Press the tip of the injector hard against the side of the child's thigh, about halfway between the hip and the knee (Figure 14B).
☐ For EpiPen and EpiPen Jr injectors, hold the injector in place for 3 seconds. Some other injectors may be held in place for up to 10 seconds. Be familiar with the manufacturer's instructions for the type of injector you are using.
☐ Pull the pen straight out. Make sure you don't put your fingers over the end that has been pressed against the child's thigh.
☐ Either the child getting the injection or the person giving the injection should rub the injection spot for about 10 seconds.
☐ Note the time of the injection. Give the pen to the emergency providers for proper disposal.
☐ If the child doesn't get better or if advanced care doesn't arrive within 10 minutes • Phone or send someone to phone 9-1-1 • Consider giving a second dose, if one is available

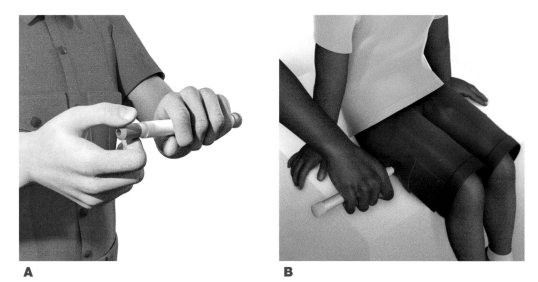

A
B

Figure 14. Using an epinephrine pen. **A**, Take off the safety cap. **B**, Press the tip of the injector hard against the side of the child's thigh, about halfway between the hip and the knee.

Dispose of the Epinephrine Pen Correctly

It's important to dispose of needles correctly so that no one gets stuck with the needle. Follow your company's disposal policy for sharp medical objects. If you don't know what to do, give the needle to someone with more advanced training.

If possible, save a sample of what caused the reaction.

Breathing Problems (Asthma)

Asthma is a disease of the air passages that carry air into the lungs. This disease can cause mild or severe narrowing of the air passages. Asthma is common in children. When severe, it can cause life-threatening breathing problems.

Some children with asthma must take daily medicine. Others take medicine only when they have asthma symptoms. Many children with asthma have an inhaler to use when they are having breathing problems (sometimes called an *asthma attack*).

Every child with asthma should have a First Aid Action Plan. If a child has an asthma attack, send another adult for the First Aid Action Plan and the child's medicines.

Step 1: Prevent

- If a child in your care has asthma, be sure that there is a First Aid Action Plan to follow in case the child develops breathing problems.
- Help the child avoid things that can trigger asthma, such as cold air and cigarette smoke.

Step 2: Protect	■ Make sure the scene is safe.
	■ Get the first aid kit.
	■ Wear PPE.

Step 3: Assess

During an asthma attack, a child may have

- Trouble breathing
- Coughing
- Tightness in the chest
- Wheezing (whistling sound)
- Fast breathing
- Difficulty speaking more than a few words at a time (severe attack)

Step 4: Act

When a child has trouble breathing, she may panic. Younger children may not be able to use their inhalers at all. You may need to assemble the inhaler and help a child use it.

How to Help a Child With Breathing Problems (Asthma)
☐ Keep calm and soothe the child. Crying can make the asthma attack worse.
☐ Follow the child's First Aid Action Plan. Send someone to get the First Aid Action Plan and the child's medicine.
☐ If the child has an inhaler, assemble it and help him use it.
☐ Phone or send someone to phone 9-1-1 if • The child has no medicine • The child does not get better after using his medicine • The child's breathing gets worse • The child becomes unresponsive
☐ Stay with the child until someone with more advanced training arrives and takes over.

Assemble and Use an Inhaler

Many children with medical conditions, such as asthma, know about their conditions and carry inhaler medicine. The medicine should make them feel better within minutes of using it.

Parts of an Inhaler

Inhalers are made up of 2 parts: the medicine canister and the mouthpiece. A spacer can be attached that makes it easier for the child with the breathing problem to inhale all of the medicine (Figure 15).

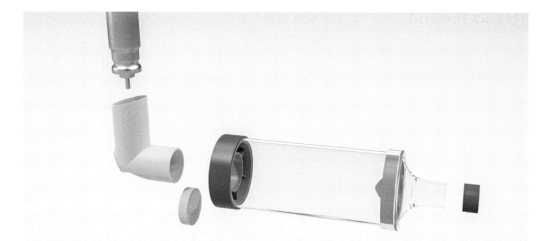

Figure 15. Parts of this inhaler are the medicine canister, mouthpiece, and spacer.

Steps to Assemble and Use an Inhaler

Follow these steps to assemble and use an inhaler:

How to Assemble and Use an Inhaler

To assemble the inhaler

☐ First, shake the medicine.

☐ Put the medicine canister into the mouthpiece.

☐ Remove the cap from the mouthpiece.

☐ Attach a spacer if there is one available and if you know how.

To help a child use an inhaler, ask him to do the following:

☐ Tilt his head back slightly and breathe out slowly.

☐ Place the inhaler or spacer in his mouth (Figure 16).

☐ Push down on the medicine canister.

☐ Breathe in very deeply and slowly.

☐ Hold his breath for about 10 seconds.

☐ Then breathe out slowly.

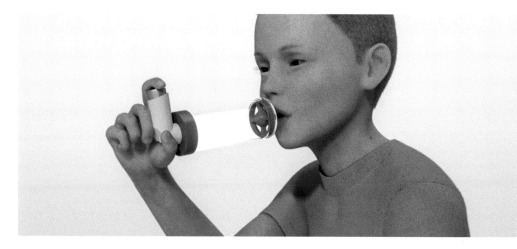

Figure 16. Using an inhaler with a spacer.

A child gets dehydrated when she doesn't have enough fluid in her body. Dehydration occurs when a child loses water or fluids through

- Heat exposure
- Too much exercise
- Vomiting, diarrhea, or fever
- Decreased fluid intake

For example, a child who loses a lot of fluid through vomiting or diarrhea and doesn't drink enough to replace the fluid she has lost can become dehydrated.

Dehydration is rarely fatal in itself, but it can lead to shock. Shock can be fatal. If you watch for and help with dehydration, you can help avoid shock. It can take a little while for an ill child to lose enough fluid to go into shock.

Step 1: Prevent

- If you help a dehydrated child, you can help prevent shock.
- Make sure a child drinks and eats enough to stay hydrated.

Step 2: Protect

- Make sure the scene is safe.
- Get the first aid kit.
- Wear PPE.

Step 3: Assess

Watch for dehydration if

- The child vomits, has diarrhea, or has a fever for 12 or more hours
- The child drinks less than usual

Signs of dehydration include

- Weakness
- Thirst
- Dry mouth
- Less urination than usual
- Less hunger than usual

Step 4: Act

Follow these steps for helping the child with dehydration:

How to Help a Child With Dehydration
☐ The best first aid for dehydration is prevention: make sure the child drinks and eats enough to stay hydrated.
☐ If you suspect a child is dehydrated or if you see signs of shock, phone or send someone to phone 9-1-1.

Diabetes and Low Blood Sugar

Diabetes is a disease that affects the level of sugar in the blood. Too much or too little sugar causes problems. Some children with diabetes take medicine, such as insulin, to maintain their sugar levels.

Children with diabetes who are not acting normally may have an illness or injury that is unrelated to diabetes. Be sure to check the child for other illnesses and injuries.

Low blood sugar can develop if a child with diabetes has

- Not eaten or is vomiting
- Not eaten enough food for the level of activity or the insulin dose
- Injected too much insulin

Step 1: Prevent

A child with diabetes probably has specific instructions from a healthcare provider on how to manage the condition. Some of the ways a child with diabetes can prevent low blood sugar include

- Keeping track of the amount of sugar in his blood
- Following a diet designed for children with diabetes
- Following the healthcare provider's directions for taking insulin

Step 2: Protect

- Make sure the scene is safe.
- Get the first aid kit.
- Wear PPE.

Step 3: Assess

Signs of low blood sugar can appear quickly and may include

- A change in behavior, such as confusion or irritability
- Sleepiness or even not responding
- Hunger, thirst, or weakness
- Sweating, pale skin color
- A seizure

Step 4: Act

Follow these steps to help a child with low blood sugar:

How to Help a Child With Low Blood Sugar
☐ Check the child's First Aid Action Plan. Follow the plan, including directions about how to check blood sugar.

If the child can't sit up and swallow

☐ Phone or have someone phone 9-1-1. Do not try to give the child anything to eat or drink.

If the child can sit up and swallow

☐ Give the child something that contains sugar to eat or drink.

☐ Have the child sit quietly or lie down.

☐ If the child does not improve within 15 minutes, phone or have someone phone 9-1-1.

Diabetic Emergency Supplies

If you are a childcare worker or teacher and have a child with diabetes in your care, make sure the First Aid Action Plan includes what to do for low blood sugar.

Children with diabetes often have emergency supplies in case of low blood sugar. Make sure the First Aid Action Plan indicates where the supplies are located. Know how to get to them quickly in an emergency.

Heat-Related Emergencies

Most heat-related emergencies are caused by vigorous exercise in a warm or hot environment. Children and infants have more trouble than adults keeping their bodies at the right temperature.

Heat-related emergencies include

- Heat cramps
- Heat exhaustion
- Heat stroke

If the child does not get first aid care for heat cramps or heat exhaustion, her condition can get worse and progress to heat stroke. Heat stroke is a life-threatening emergency.

Heat Cramps

Heat cramps are painful muscle spasms. They usually occur in the calves, arms, stomach muscles, and back.

Step 1: Prevent

- Heat cramps are caused by dehydration. Make sure the child drinks water or sports drinks before and during outside play in hot weather.
- Avoid outside play when temperatures are very hot.
- See "Heat Exhaustion" for more steps in preventing heat-related illness.

Step 2: Protect

- Make sure the scene is safe.
- Get the first aid kit.
- Wear PPE.

Step 3: Assess

Signs of heat cramps are

- Muscle cramps
- Sweating
- Headache

Heat cramps are a sign that the child needs first aid care. Heat-related problems can get worse and be life threatening.

Step 4: Act

Follow these steps to help a child with heat cramps:

How to Help a Child With Heat Cramps
☐ Have the child rest and cool off.
☐ Have the child drink something with sugar and electrolytes, such as a sports drink or juice. Offer water if these aren't available.
☐ If the child can tolerate it, apply a bag with ice and water wrapped in a towel to the cramping area for up to 20 minutes.

Although heat exhaustion is not life threatening, it can quickly become heat stroke. Heat stroke is life threatening. Heat exhaustion is caused by dehydration. It often occurs when a child exercises in the heat and sweats a lot.

Step 1: Prevent

- Children should stay hydrated before and after exercise.
- During exercise, children should drink water or sports drinks often to stay hydrated.
- Children should wear lightweight, light-colored clothes when exercising in the sun or heat.
- If it's very hot or humid, children should avoid exercising outdoors.
- Children should exercise during cooler times of the day.
- Carefully watch children who aren't fit or aren't used to exercising in the heat.
- If a child looks ill or not normal (not like himself), have him stop exercising. Check for signs of heat exhaustion or heat stroke.

Step 2: Protect

- Make sure the scene is safe.
- Get the first aid kit.
- Wear PPE.

Step 3: Assess

Look for the following signs of heat exhaustion:

- Sweating
- Nausea
- Dizziness
- Vomiting
- Muscle cramps
- Feeling faint or fatigued

Step 4: Act

Follow these steps to help a child with heat exhaustion:

How to Help a Child With Heat Exhaustion
☐ Phone or send someone to phone 9-1-1.
☐ Have the child lie down in a cool place.
☐ Remove as much of the child's clothing as possible.
☐ Cool the child with a cool (but not ice-cold) water spray. If cool water spray is not available, place cool damp cloths on the neck, armpit, and groin area.
☐ If the child is responsive and can drink, have the child drink something that contains sugar and electrolytes, such as juice or a sports drink. Offer water if these aren't available.

Heat Stroke

Heat-related conditions can progress quickly if not recognized and treated. Heat stroke is a dangerous condition that is life threatening.

It's important to begin cooling a child who might have heat stroke immediately—every minute counts. If you can't put the child into cool (but not ice-cold) water up to his neck, try to cool him with a cool water spray.

If the child starts behaving normally again, stop cooling him. If you cool the child too much, it can lead to low body temperature.

Step 1: Prevent

- Follow the same prevention steps as for heat exhaustion.
- Giving first aid to a child who has heat exhaustion will help keep heat exhaustion from becoming heat stroke.
- Never leave a child or infant in a hot car. See "Car Safety: Preventing Injury" in the Child and Infant Safety Checklist.

Step 2: Protect

- Make sure the scene is safe.
- Get the first aid kit and AED.
- Wear PPE.

Step 3: Assess

Look for the following signs of heat stroke:

- Confusion or unresponsiveness
- Passing out
- Dizziness
- Seizure
- Feeling faint or fatigued
- Nausea, vomiting
- Muscle cramps

Step 4: Act

Follow these steps to help a child with heat stroke:

How to Help a Child With Heat Stroke
☐ Phone or send someone to phone 9-1-1.
☐ Put the child in cool (but not ice-cold) water up to his neck if possible, or spray him with cool water.
☐ Give CPR if the child doesn't respond and is not breathing or is only gasping.

Cold-Related Emergencies

Cold-related emergencies may involve the whole body or only part of the body.

- Cold injury to the whole body is called *low body temperature* or *hypothermia.*
- Cold injury to part of the body is called *frostbite.*

Low Body Temperature

Cold injury to the whole body is called *low body temperature* or *hypothermia.* Hypothermia occurs when body temperature falls. This is a serious condition that can cause death.

Here are some key points to remember about hypothermia:

- A child can develop hypothermia even when the temperature is above freezing. For example, a child can get hypothermia from walking in the rain and wind without a jacket.
- Very small children and infants can easily develop hypothermia.
- Shivering protects the body by producing heat. Shivering stops when the body becomes very cold.

Step 1: Prevent	■ Make sure children wear appropriate clothing in cold weather.
	■ Watch small children closely if they are in very cold weather to make sure they stay warm and dry.

Step 2: Protect	■ Make sure the scene is safe.
	■ Get the first aid kit and AED.
	■ Wear PPE.

Step 3: Assess

Look for signs of hypothermia, which include

■ Skin that's cool to the touch

■ Shivering, which stops when the body temperature is very low

■ Confusion or drowsiness

■ Personality changes

■ Sleepiness and lack of concern about this condition

■ Stiff, rigid muscles while the skin becomes ice-cold and blue

■ Slowed breathing

As the child's body temperature continues to drop, it may be hard to tell if the child is breathing. The child may become unresponsive and even appear to be dead.

Step 4: Act

Follow these steps to help a child with low body temperature:

How to Help a Child With Low Body Temperature
☐ Get the child out of the cold.
☐ Phone or send someone to phone 9-1-1 if you suspect hypothermia.
☐ Remove wet clothing, pat the child dry, and cover with a blanket.
☐ Put dry clothes on the child.   • Cover the body and head, but not the face, with blankets, towels, or even newspapers.
☐ Remain with the child until someone with more advanced training arrives and takes over.
☐ Give CPR if the child doesn't respond and is not breathing or is only gasping.

Frostbite affects parts of the body that are exposed to the cold, such as the fingers, toes, nose, and ears.

Frostbite typically occurs outside in cold weather. But it can also occur inside when children without gloves handle extremely cold materials.

Step 1: Prevent

- Make sure children wear appropriate clothing in cold weather.
- Watch small children closely if they are in very cold weather to make sure they stay warm.

Step 2: Protect

- Make sure the scene is safe.
- Get the first aid kit.
- Wear PPE.

Step 3: Assess

The signs of frostbite include the following:

- The skin over the frostbitten area is white, waxy, or grayish-yellow.
- The frostbitten area is cold and numb.
- The frostbitten area is hard, and the skin doesn't move when you push it.

Step 4: Act

Follow these steps to help a child with frostbite:

How to Help a Child With Frostbite
☐ Move the child to a warm place.
☐ Phone or send someone to phone 9-1-1 and get the first aid kit.
☐ Remove tight clothing and jewelry from the frostbitten part.
☐ Remove wet clothing and pat the body dry.
☐ Put dry clothes on the child and cover him with a blanket.

Caution

These are things you *should not do* for frostbite:

- Do not try to thaw the frozen part if you think there may be a chance that it will freeze again before the child can get to medical care.
- Do not rub the frostbitten area because it can cause damage. If you need to touch the area, do so gently.

Drowning is a leading cause of preventable death in children younger than 15 years old. Children are very attracted to water; they can drown if they enter the water without adult supervision.

Young children can drown in very shallow water, such as a 5-gallon bucket or in the bathtub.

Step 1: Prevent

- Do not leave a child alone around any water.
  - The head of a small child or an infant or is very heavy compared with the rest of his body.
  - A small child or infant can lean over and fall into a bucket, toilet, or small container. He may not be able to lift his head out of the water.
- Swimming pools, creeks, fountains, lakes, and rivers are very appealing to most children. It is important to closely watch all children near pools or other bodies of water.
  - Any child or infant can drown, even if he knows how to swim.
  - Always stay within reach of a child when near a body of water.
  - Use life jackets when appropriate.
- See the Child and Infant Safety Checklist for more ways to prevent drowning.

Step 2: Protect

- Make sure the scene is safe.
- Get the first aid kit and AED.
- Wear PPE.

Step 3: Assess

If the child is wet and not breathing, the child may have drowned.

Step 4: Act

If you see a child who may be drowning, follow these steps:

How to Help a Child Who Is Drowning
☐ If the child is under water, get her out safely. Remove the child from the water.
☐ Give CPR if the child doesn't respond and is not breathing or only gasping.
☐ If the child doesn't need CPR, remove wet clothing and wrap her in dry blankets.
☐ Continue to check if the child needs CPR.

Children who drown in cold water may have no breathing, cold and blue skin, and stiff muscles. Even if the child appears dead, start CPR right away. Continue until someone with more advanced training arrives and takes over.

Illnesses and Injuries: Group A Review Questions

Question	Your Notes
1. What can stop most severe bleeding? a. Putting on gloves b. Putting direct pressure on the wound c. Applying an antibiotic cream d. Having the child lie down	
2. Which of the following should be used as a dressing? a. A clean cloth b. A cold pack c. A dirty cloth d. A piece of tape	
3. Shock happens when a child has lost too much blood or water. True False	
4. Which of the following is true of an epinephrine pen injection? a. It can be given through clothes or on bare skin. b. It should be used for every child with a rash. c. It can only be given through bare skin. d. It is always given in the side of the arm.	
5. When a child has an asthma attack, what should you do? a. Give him something with sugar to drink. b. Leave him alone until his breathing gets better. c. Help the child use his prescription medicine. d. Give him thrusts above the belly button.	

(continued)

Question	Your Notes
6. If a child with low blood sugar is able to sit up and swallow, give her something containing sugar to eat or drink. True False	

7. Which of the following is true of heat stroke?
 	
  a. Heat stroke can quickly turn into heat exhaustion.
 	
  b. Heat stroke is not dangerous.
 	
  c. Heat stroke can be caused by exercising outside when the weather is very warm or hot.
 	
  d. Heat stroke should be treated with warm water.	

8. How can a child get hypothermia (low body temperature)?
 	
  a. From walking in rain and wind without a jacket
 	
  b. On a hot, sunny day
 	
  c. When she doesn't have enough sugar in her blood
 	
  d. After a seizure	

9. In which of the following can a young child drown?
 	
  a. A 5-gallon bucket
 	
  b. A toilet
 	
  c. A bathtub
 	
  d. All of the above	

Answers: 1. b, 2. a, 3. True, 4. a, 5. c, 6. True, 7. c, 8. a, 9. d

Part 3: Illnesses and Injuries: Group B

Group B includes illnesses and injuries that you should be familiar with. Some may not be as urgent, but they still have the potential to become serious. The most important actions that you can take are to recognize that something is wrong and begin first aid care.

Topics Covered

Topics covered in this part are

- Amputations
- Bites and stings
- Broken bones, sprains, and bruises
- Eye injuries
- Bleeding from the nose
- Fainting
- Fever
- Head, neck, and spinal injuries
- Penetrating and puncturing injuries
- Poison emergencies
- Seizure
- Mouth and cheek injuries
- Tooth injuries
- Splinters

As you read and study this part, pay particular attention to this skill that you may be asked to demonstrate during the course:

Skill • Splinting (optional)

Amputations

One injury that may seem overwhelming is traumatic amputation.

Amputation occurs when any part of the body is cut or torn off. It may be possible to reattach certain body parts. So it's important to know what to do. First, stop bleeding by applying pressure. You may need to use a tourniquet if bleeding is severe. Then protect the amputated part.

You can preserve a detached body part at room temperature, but it will be in better condition to be reattached if you keep it cool.

Step 1: Prevent Use the Child and Infant Safety Checklist to prevent injuries that may lead to amputation.

Step 2: Protect
- Make sure the scene is safe.
- Get the first aid kit.
- Wear PPE.

Step 3: Assess Find the part of the body that has been amputated.

Step 4: Act Follow these steps to protect an amputated part:

First Aid Steps for an Amputation
☐ Phone or send someone to phone 9-1-1.
☐ Stop the bleeding from the injured area with pressure. You may have to press for a long time with very firm pressure to stop the bleeding.
☐ If you find the amputated part, follow "How to Protect an Amputated Part" below.
☐ Stay with the injured child until someone with more advanced training arrives and takes over.

Follow these steps when a part of the body has been amputated:

How to Protect an Amputated Part
☐ Rinse the amputated part with clean water (Figure 17A).
☐ Cover it with a clean dressing.
☐ Place it in a watertight plastic bag (Figure 17B).
☐ Place the bag in another container with ice or ice and water (Figure 17C). Label it with the injured child's name, the date, and the time.
☐ Make sure the body part gets to the hospital with the injured child.
Remember: Do not place the amputated body part directly on ice because extreme cold can injure it. Always put something in between a body part and the ice and water.

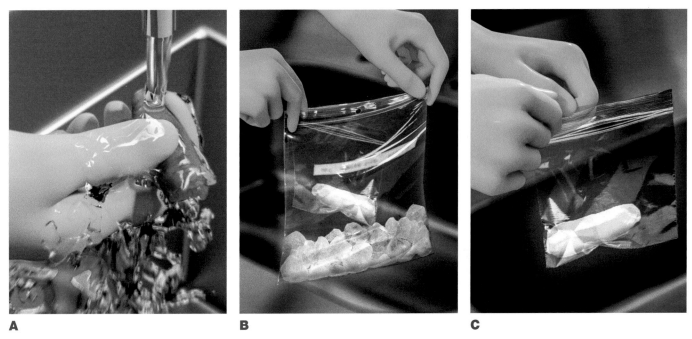

A   B   C

Figure 17. A, If you can find the amputated part, rinse it with clean water. **B**, If it will fit, place the wrapped part in a watertight plastic bag. **C**, Place that bag in another labeled bag that contains ice or ice and water.

Bites and Stings

Bites and stings are common injuries to children. The risk of many animal bites and insect bites and stings will vary according to location and time of year. For example, scorpions are found in dry climates. Ticks are a problem in wooded areas. Marine animals live in or near the ocean.

Be familiar with the bites and stings that occur most often in your area. Be prepared to give first aid care.

Human and Animal Bites

Young, preschool-aged children sometimes bite each other. Some young children will bite others to show their feelings. Most children stop biting when they grow older.

Animal bites are less common and often can be prevented. Unfortunately, when they do occur, animal bites can be serious.

When a bite breaks the skin, the wound can bleed. It may become infected from the germs in the child's or animal's mouth. Bites that do not break the skin usually are not serious.

Not only is the bite a concern, there can be a risk of rabies from dogs or wild animals. Rabies in wild animals is most often reported in raccoons, skunks, and bats. Dogs bitten by infected animals can become infected.

| **Step 1: Prevent** | ▪ Take precautions to protect children from bites. See the Child and Infant Safety Checklist. |
| | ▪ Some bites get infected. You can help prevent this by washing small wounds well as soon as possible. |

Step 2: Protect	▪ Make sure the scene is safe.
	▪ Stay away from any animal that acts strangely.
	▪ Get the first aid kit.
	▪ Wear PPE.

| **Step 3: Assess** | Find where the child was bitten. |

Step 4: Act

Follow these steps to help a child with a human or animal bite:

How to Help a Child With an Animal or Human Bite

☐ Wash the wound with plenty of soap and water.

☐ Stop any bleeding with pressure or bandages.

☐ If there is a bruise or swelling, place a bag of ice and water wrapped in a towel on the bite for up to 20 minutes.

☐ For all bites that break the skin, contact a healthcare provider as soon as possible.

Risk of Rabies

Animals that may carry rabies include a cat, dog, skunk, raccoon, fox, bat, or other wild animal. Always contact a healthcare provider right away for any bite that breaks the skin.

Also, because of the risk of rabies, anyone who has had direct contact with a bat or has been alone in a room with a bat should contact a healthcare provider as soon as possible.

Snakebites

Bites from poisonous snakes are a first aid emergency. If a child has been bitten by a snake, try to identify the type of snake. This can help with treatment. Sometimes you can tell what type of snake it is from the color or bite mark. But if you're not sure, assume that the snake is poisonous.

Step 1: Prevent	■ Teach children to leave snakes alone and to stay away from snakes. Teach them to tell an adult when they see a snake.
	■ Keep outdoor play areas away from places where snakes can live. This includes tall grass or piles of rock or firewood.
	■ Teach children not to reach into places where snakes may hide.

Step 2: Protect	■ Make sure the scene is safe.
	■ Be very careful around any snake, even if it's wounded. Back away and go around the snake.
	■ If a snake has been hurt or killed, don't handle it. A snake can bite even when badly hurt or close to death.
	■ If a snake needs to be moved, use a long-handled shovel. If you don't need to move it, leave it alone.
	■ Get the first aid kit.
	■ Wear PPE.

Step 3: Assess	Look for these signs that a snakebite is poisonous. They include
	■ Pain at the bite area that keeps getting worse
	■ Swelling of the bite area
	■ Nausea, vomiting, sweating, or weakness

Step 4: Act	Follow these steps to help a child who has been bitten by a snake:

How to Help a Child With a Snakebite
☐ Ask another adult to move any other people away from the area. Phone or send someone to phone 9-1-1.
☐ Ask the injured child to stay still and calm. Tell him to avoid moving the part of the body that was bitten.
☐ Remove any tight clothing and jewelry.
☐ Gently wash the area with running water and soap.
☐ Keep the child still and calm until someone with more advanced training arrives and takes over.

Other First Aid for Snakebites	Some people have heard other ways to give first aid for a snakebite, such as sucking out poison. Don't do that. Follow the steps listed in the workbook to give first aid care for a snakebite.

Usually insect bites and stings cause only mild pain, itching, and swelling at the bite. However, some insect bites can be serious and even fatal if

- Poison (venom) is injected into the child from the bite or sting
- The child has a severe allergic reaction to the bite or sting

Bees are the only insects that leave behind their stingers. If a child gets stung by a bee, look for the stinger and remove it.

Step 1: Prevent

Take the following steps to prevent insect bites and stings:

- Keep children from bothering insects.
- Use insect repellent that is approved for use on children.
- If you know a child has a severe allergy to an insect or bee sting, keep his epinephrine pen close by at all times. This is especially important when the child is outdoors.
- Have children wear light-colored clothing when they are in areas where insects are likely to be. Their clothing should cover their arms and legs.
- Keep flowering plants and gardens away from areas where children play.
- Put outdoor toys away so spiders and insects can't hide inside them.

Step 2: Protect

- Make sure the scene is safe.
- Get the first aid kit.
- Wear PPE.

Step 3: Assess

Find the area that has been bitten or stung. Try to figure out if the bite is poisonous or not.

The bite or sting of insects that aren't poisonous can cause mild signs of redness and itching at the bite area. However, the bite of a poisonous spider or scorpion can cause a child to become ill.

Signs of poisonous spider and scorpion bites are

- Severe pain at the site of the bite or sting
- Muscle cramps
- Headache
- Fever
- Vomiting
- Breathing problems
- Seizures
- Unresponsiveness

Step 4: Act

Take first aid steps for a child with an insect bite or sting.

Actions for a Bite or Sting From a Nonpoisonous Insect

Follow these steps to help a child with a bite or sting:

How to Help a Child With a Bite or Sting
☐ If the child was stung by a bee, scrape the stinger and venom sac away with something hard and dull that won't squeeze it—like the edge of a credit card or photo ID card. (Squeezing the venom sac can release more poison.)
☐ Wash the sting or bite area with running water and soap.
☐ Put a bag of ice and water wrapped in a towel over the area for up to 20 minutes.
☐ Watch the child for at least 30 minutes for signs of a severe allergic reaction. Be prepared to use the child's epinephrine pen if needed.

Severe Allergic Reactions to Bee Stings

Children who have had severe allergic reactions to an insect bite or sting usually have an epinephrine pen and know how to use it. They often wear medical identification jewelry.

If a child with a known allergy to bees has an insect bite or sting (even if you're not sure the child was stung by a bee), get the first aid kit and the child's epinephrine pen. If the child develops a severe allergic reaction, phone or send someone to phone 9-1-1. Use the skills you learned earlier to help the child inject epinephrine by using her epinephrine pen. Be prepared to help the child give a second injection if needed.

Actions for a Bite or Sting From a Poisonous Spider or Scorpion

Follow these steps if you know that a child has been bitten or stung by a poisonous spider or scorpion. Also, follow these steps if the child has any of the signs that a bite or sting might be from a poisonous spider or scorpion:

How to Help a Child With a Bite or Sting From a Poisonous Spider or Scorpion
☐ Phone or send someone to phone 9-1-1.
☐ Wash the bite with lots of running water and soap.
☐ Put a bag of ice and water wrapped in a towel on the bite or sting.
☐ Keep the child still and calm until someone with more advanced training arrives and takes over.

Ticks are found on animals and in wooded areas. They attach themselves to exposed body parts. Many ticks are harmless but some carry serious diseases.

If you find a tick, remove it as soon as possible. The longer the tick stays attached to a child, the greater the child's chance of catching a disease.

Step 1: Prevent

- Wear proper clothing.
  - Children should wear light-colored clothing so you can see the tick more easily later.
  - Clothing should cover a child's arms and legs. Tuck pants into the child's socks or boots.
- Take precautions in wooded or brushy areas.
  - Children should avoid wooded areas with dead leaves and other debris. They also should avoid brushy areas with high grass. These areas are home to many insects, especially ticks.
  - Children should stay on the trails when walking through wooded or brushy areas.
- Use insect repellent safely.
  - Insect repellent products containing DEET may be used on children over 2 months old if the label says it is safe for use on children.
  - Select a repellant that contains no more than 30% DEET.
  - Use DEET products only on infants older than 2 months.
  - Do not use sunscreen containing DEET. This is because the DEET can build up when you reapply sunscreen frequently.
  - Do not use products containing lemon eucalyptus oil on children younger than 3 years old.
- Be careful when using insect repellant.
  - Don't spray the repellant on the child. Instead, apply to your own hands. Then rub it on the child.
  - Avoid putting repellant on children's hands or around the eyes. Also don't put repellant on cut or irritated skin.
  - Do not allow children to handle insect repellents.
  - After returning indoors, wash the child's treated skin or bathe the child.
  - Wash clothes exposed to insect repellants with soap and water.

Step 2: Protect

- Make sure the scene is safe.
- Get the first aid kit.
- Wear PPE.
- Check the child's hair and skin after being in areas where ticks are found.

Step 3: Assess

- Find the tick bite.

Step 4: Act   Follow these steps to help a child with a tick bite:

How to Help a Child With a Tick Bite
☐ Use tweezers to grab the tick by its mouth or head, as close to the skin as possible.
☐ Try to avoid pinching the tick.
☐ Lift the tick straight out. If you lift the tick until the child's skin tents and wait for several seconds, the tick may let go.
☐ Place the tick in a plastic bag so the caregiver can take it to the healthcare provider if needed.
☐ Wash the bite with running water and soap.
☐ See a healthcare provider if the child is in a region of the country where tick-borne diseases occur.

Other First Aid for Tick Bites   Some people have heard about other ways to remove a tick. The correct way to remove a tick is to follow the steps in this workbook.

Marine Bites and Stings

You have learned that it's important to be aware of ticks and other insects and animals when you're in the wilderness. It's just as important to be aware of marine fish and animals when at the beach or swimming in the ocean.

Bites and stings from jellyfish, stingrays, or stonefish can cause pain, swelling, redness, or bleeding. Some marine bites and stings can be serious. They can even be fatal if a child has a severe allergic reaction to the sting or the venom.

Step 1: Prevent
- At the beach, watch for signs that warn you about dangerous jellyfish or other marine life.
- Even dead marine animals can sting. Avoid touching them with bare hands or skin.

Step 2: Protect
- Make sure the scene is safe.
- Get the first aid kit.
- Wear PPE.
- Try to avoid touching a biting or stinging marine animal. But if you must, use something to protect your bare skin.

Step 3: Assess

The following are signs of a poisonous marine bite or sting:

- Chest pain
- Cramps
- Fever
- Weakness, faintness, or dizziness
- Nausea or vomiting
- Numbness or trouble moving parts of the body
- Severe pain and swelling
- Color changes of the skin in the area bitten or stung

Step 4: Act

Follow these steps to help a child with a marine bite or sting:

How to Help a Child With a Marine Bite or Sting

- ☐ Keep the injured child quiet and still.

- ☐ Wipe off stingers or tentacles with a gloved hand or towel.

- ☐ If the sting is from a jellyfish, rinse the injured area for at least 30 seconds with lots of vinegar. If vinegar is not available, use a baking soda and water solution instead.

- ☐ Put the part of the body that was stung in hot water. You may also have the child take a shower with water as hot as he can bear, for at least 20 minutes or as long as pain persists. If hot water is not available, apply dry hot or cold packs for up to 20 minutes instead.

- ☐ Phone or send someone to phone 9-1-1 if
  - A child has been bitten or stung by a marine animal and has signs of a severe allergic reaction
  - A child was bitten or stung in an area known to have poisonous marine animals

- ☐ For all bites and stings that break the skin, contact a healthcare provider as soon as possible.

Broken Bones, Sprains, and Bruises

Broken bones, sprains, and bruises are common first aid emergencies. Joint sprains happen when joints move in directions they're not supposed to. A child may get a bruise if he is hit or runs into a hard object. Bruises happen when blood collects under the skin. They can appear as red or black-and-blue spots.

It is hard to tell whether a bone is broken or a joint is sprained without an x-ray. You will give the same first aid care for both injuries.

Step 1: Prevent	Use the Child and Infant Safety Checklist to help prevent injuries that may lead to broken bones, sprains, and bruises.

Step 2: Protect	<ul><li>Make sure the scene is safe.</li><li>Get the first aid kit.</li><li>Wear PPE.</li><li>Remove jewelry from the injured area if possible.</li></ul>

Step 3: Assess	Assess the injured area. Look for broken bones or sprains. Signs include <ul><li>Swelling</li><li>Pain</li><li>Not being able to move the injured part</li><li>A joint turning slightly blue</li></ul>

Step 4: Act

Follow these steps to help a child with a broken bone, sprain, or bruise:

How to Help a Child With a Broken Bone, Sprain, or Bruise

☐ Cover any open wound with a clean dressing.

☐ Put a towel on top of the injured body part. Place a bag filled with ice and water* on top of the towel over the injured area (Figure 18). Keep the ice in place for up to 20 minutes.

☐ Phone or send someone to phone 9-1-1 if
- There is a large open wound
- The injured body part is abnormally bent
- You're not sure what to do

☐ If it hurts, the child should avoid using the injured body part until checked by a healthcare provider.

*If ice is not available, you can use a bag of frozen vegetables. Also, you may use a cold pack. But it will not be as cold and may not work as well as ice and water.

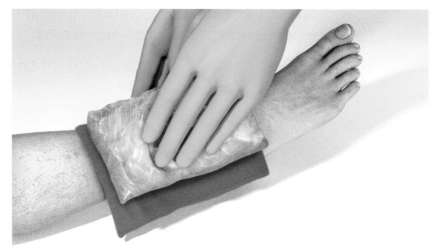

Figure 18. Put a plastic bag filled with ice and water on the injured area with a towel between the ice bag and the skin.

Splinting

A splint keeps an injured body part from moving (Figure 19). If a broken bone has come through the skin or is bent, it shouldn't be straightened. The injury needs to be protected until someone with more advanced training arrives and takes over.

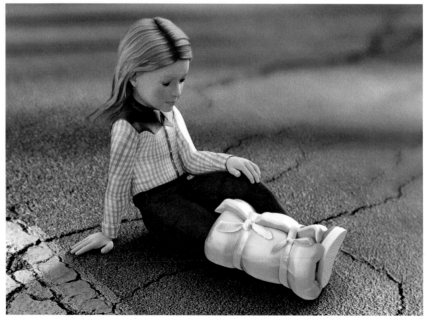

Figure 19. A splint keeps an injured body part from moving.

Caution

If the injured part is bleeding, apply direct pressure to stop the bleeding. Put a dressing on the wound before applying the splint.

Leave bent and deformed body parts in their bent or deformed positions as you apply the splint. If a broken bone has come through the skin, cover the wound with a clean dressing. Splint as needed.

Phone or send someone to phone 9-1-1 if

- There is a large open wound
- The injured part is abnormally bent
- You're not sure what to do

Step 1: Prevent

Use the Child and Infant Safety Checklist to help prevent injuries that may lead to broken bones.

Step 2: Protect

- Make sure the scene is safe.
- Get the first aid kit.
- Wear PPE.

Step 3: Assess

Assess the need for a splint. Most of the time, splints are applied by a healthcare provider. However, sometimes you may need to splint an arm or a leg. For example, if you are hiking in the wilderness and a child breaks his arm, you may need to apply a splint. A splint will help keep the injury from getting worse until the child can get medical care.

Step 4: Act

Follow these steps to apply a splint:

How to Apply a Splint

☐ Find an object that you can use to keep the injured arm or leg from moving.

☐ Rolled-up towels, magazines, and pieces of wood can be used as splints. Splint in a way to reduce pain and limit further injury. The splint should be longer than the injured area. It should support the joints above and below the injury.

☐ After covering any broken skin with a clean or sterile cloth, tie or tape the splint to the injured limb so that it supports the injured area (Figure 20).

☐ Use tape, gauze, or cloth to secure it. It should fit snugly but not cut off circulation.

☐ If you're using a hard splint, like wood, make sure you pad it with something soft, like clothing or a towel.

☐ Keep the limb still until the injured child can be seen by a healthcare provider.

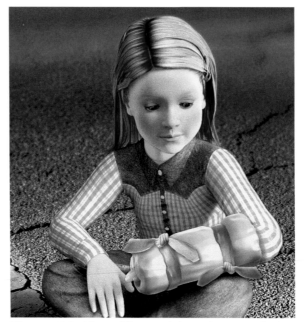

Figure 20. Use stiff material, such as a rolled-up magazine, to splint injured body parts.

How to Self-Splint an Arm

If you don't have anything to use as a splint, the child can use her other arm to hold the injured one in place. Follow these steps to self-splint an arm:

How to Self-Splint an Arm

☐ Have the injured child place her hand across her chest and hold it in place with her other arm.

Eye injuries in children can occur at home, at school, or during play. Some common eye injuries in children happen from a

- Direct hit or punch to the eye or to the side of the head
- Direct hit from a ball or other object
- High-speed object (such as a BB gun pellet)
- Stick or other sharp object that punctures the eye
- Small object, such as a piece of dirt, that gets in the eye

Step 1: Prevent

Some ways that you can prevent eye injury are the following:

- Be sure that children wear proper eye protection when playing sports.
- Monitor toys with eye safety in mind.
- Keep objects that can cause eye injury away from children. Or supervise children very closely if they use these objects. Examples of objects that can cause eye injury are rubber bands and pointed scissors.
- Keep chemicals and sprays out of reach.

Step 2: Protect

- Make sure the scene is safe.
- Get the first aid kit.
- Wear PPE.

Step 3: Assess

Assess the eye for signs of injury, such as

- Pain
- Trouble seeing
- Bruising
- Bleeding
- Redness, swelling

Step 4: Act

Follow these steps to help a child with an eye injury:

How to Help a Child With an Eye Injury
☐ If something small like sand gets in a child's eye, rinse with lots of running water.

☐ Phone or send someone to phone 9-1-1 if the
  - Object doesn't come out
  - Child complains about extreme pain
  - Child still has trouble seeing

☐ Tell the child to keep his eyes closed until someone with more advanced training arrives and takes over.

Bleeding From the Nose

Nosebleeds are common in children. Some reasons for nosebleeds are injury, irritation, and picking the nose.

Step 1: Prevent

Use the Child and Infant Safety Checklist to help prevent injuries that lead to bleeding from the nose.

Step 2: Protect

- Make sure the scene is safe.
- Get the first aid kit.
- Wear PPE.

Step 3: Assess

Assess the child to find the source of the bleeding.

Step 4: Act

To stop a nosebleed, apply pressure. Follow these steps:

How to Help a Child With a Nosebleed
☐ Have the child sit and lean forward.
☐ Pinch the soft part of the nose on both sides (Figure 21) with a clean dressing.
☐ Place constant pressure on the nostrils for a few minutes until the bleeding stops. If bleeding continues, press harder.

☐ Phone or send someone to phone 9-1-1 if
  • You can't stop the bleeding in about 15 minutes
  • The bleeding is heavy, such as gushing blood
  • The injured child has trouble breathing

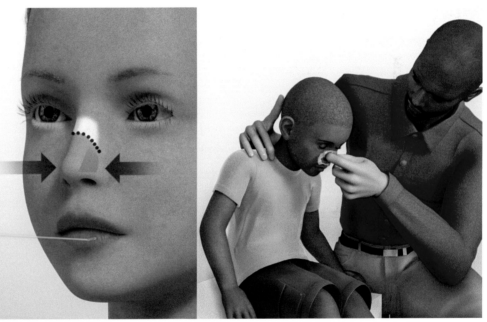

Figure 21. Press on both sides of the nostrils. Have the child lean forward.

First Aid Myth

A child with a nosebleed should lean forward (not backward). Leaning backward will not help stop the bleeding. You will see less blood when a child tilts his head back. This is because the blood drains down the child's throat. Swallowed blood can lead to vomiting.

Fainting is when a child briefly stops responding for a short period of time. This period of time is usually less than a minute. After that, the child seems fine. Often, a child who faints gets dizzy and then becomes unresponsive for a short period.

Fainting may occur when a child

- Stands without moving for a long time, especially if it's hot
- Has a heart condition
- Suddenly stands after squatting or bending down
- Receives bad news

Step 1: Prevent

If a child feels dizzy or weak, move her to a safe place. If it's hot outside and the child is alert, it may help to give the child something cool to drink.

Step 2: Protect

- Make sure the scene is safe.
- Get the first aid kit.
- Wear PPE.

Step 3: Assess

A child who is about to faint may feel dizzy, light-headed, and weak.

Step 4: Act

Follow these steps if a child is dizzy but still responds:

How to Help a Child Who May Faint
☐ Help the child lie flat on the floor.
☐ Phone or send someone to phone 9-1-1 if the child doesn't improve or becomes unresponsive.
☐ Give CPR if the child doesn't respond and is not breathing or only gasping.

Follow these steps if a child faints and then starts to respond:

How to Help a Child Who Has Fainted and Is Responsive
☐ Ask the child to continue to lie flat on the floor until he can sit up and feels normal.
☐ If the child fell, look for injuries caused by the fall.
☐ If the child feels normal, contact a healthcare provider.
☐ If the child doesn't improve or stops responding again,   • Phone or send someone to phone 9-1-1   • Give CPR if the child is not responsive and is not breathing or only gasping

Fever

Fever is a high body temperature. It's the body's natural way of fighting illness. Fever can be caused by an illness or infection.

Some fevers are low-grade and don't need first aid. Some children with a fever may have a seizure.

Use a thermometer that is not made of glass to take the child's temperature. Glass can break and hurt the child. You can take the child's temperature at several parts of the body. These places are recommended:

- In the armpit
- Under the tongue
- In the ear (using a thermometer made for use in the ear)
- Across the forehead

Step 1: Prevent

You can't prevent fevers. Washing hands can help prevent illnesses from spreading.

Step 2: Protect

Keep a child with fever away from other children.

Step 3: Assess

If the child feels hot or if you suspect a child has a fever, check the child's temperature.

Step 4: Act

Follow these steps to help a child with a fever:

How to Help a Child With a Fever
☐ Contact the parent, caregiver, or healthcare provider if a child has a fever.
☐ Give medicine to reduce fever only if the child's parent, caregiver, or healthcare provider tells you to give it and approves the medicine you are giving.
☐ Move the sick child away from any other children to help prevent other children from becoming ill.
☐ Phone or send someone to phone 9-1-1 if the child • Has a seizure • Has trouble breathing • Shows signs of shock or dehydration • Is hard to wake up

Aspirin Can Be Dangerous for Children

Giving aspirin to children can be very dangerous and can lead to Reye's Syndrome. Only give aspirin if a healthcare provider specifically tells you to. Aspirin is different from ibuprofen or acetaminophen.

Head, Neck, and Spinal Injuries

With any kind of head, neck, or spinal injury, be cautious about moving an injured child.

Suspect a head, neck, or spinal injury if the child

- Fell from a height
- Was injured by a strong blow to the head
- Was injured while diving
- Was involved in a car crash
- Was riding a bicycle or motorbike involved in a crash, especially if the helmet broke in the crash or the child was not wearing a helmet.

Signs of a Head Injury

If you think a child has a serious head injury, phone or send someone to phone 9-1-1. Suspect a head injury if an injured child

- Does not respond or only moans
- Acts sleepy or confused
- Vomits
- Has trouble seeing, walking, or moving any part of the body
- Has a seizure

A child should be evaluated by a healthcare or EMS provider as soon as possible if his signs and symptoms get worse. Other reasons for immediate evaluation are a change in responsiveness or another cause for concern.

If the child becomes unresponsive, be sure that someone has phoned 9-1-1. Give CPR if the child is not responding and is not breathing or only gasping.

A child with signs of a head injury should not play sports, ride a bike, or do similar activities until a healthcare provider says it's OK.

Concussion

A concussion is a type of head injury. Concussions usually happen because of falls, motor vehicle crashes, and sports injuries. A concussion may occur when the head or body is hit so hard that the brain moves inside the skull.

Possible signs of concussion are

- Feeling stunned or dazed
- Confusion
- Headache
- Nausea or vomiting
- Dizziness, unsteadiness, difficulty in balance
- Double vision or flashing lights
- Loss of memory of events that happened before or after the injury

If a child has a head injury and any of these signs, contact a healthcare provider right away. Phone or send someone to phone 9-1-1 if a child with a head injury

- Loses consciousness
- Has a change in level of consciousness—for example, becomes sleepier or more irritable
- Has a progression of signs—for example, is alert at first and then becomes confused, speaks clearly at first and then begins to mumble, or is sleepy and gets sleepier instead of waking up
- Has other causes for concern

Spinal Injury

If a child falls, an injury to the spine is possible. The bones of the spine protect the spinal cord. The spinal cord carries messages between the brain and the body.

If the spine is damaged, the spinal cord may be injured. The child may not be able to move her legs or arms. She may lose feeling in parts of the body.

Suspect possible spinal damage if the child

- Was in a car or bicycle crash
- Has fallen from a height
- Has tingling or is weak in the hands and feet
- Has pain or tenderness in the neck or back
- Appears "drunk" or not fully alert
- Has other painful injuries, especially of the head or neck

Step 1: Prevent

Falls are a leading cause of head, neck, and spinal injuries. Use the Child and Infant Safety Checklist to help keep a child safe from falls.

Step 2: Protect

- Make sure the scene is safe.
- Get the first aid kit and AED.
- Wear PPE.
- Try not to move the child. If you must move the child, use caution.

Caution

When a child has a spinal injury, *do not twist or turn the head or neck* unless it's necessary to do any of the following:

- Turn the child faceup to give CPR
- Move the child out of danger
- Reposition the child because of breathing problems, vomiting, or fluids in the mouth

Step 3: Assess

Check an injured child for signs of head injury, concussion, and spinal injury (see above).

Step 4: Act

Follow these steps to help a child with a head, neck, or spinal injury:

How to Help a Child With a Possible Head, Neck, or Spinal Injury
☐ Phone or send someone to phone 9-1-1 and get the first aid kit and the AED.
☐ Have the child remain as still as possible. Wait for someone with more advanced training to arrive and take over.
☐ ***Do not twist or turn the child's head or neck*** unless absolutely necessary. See "Caution" under "Step 2: Protect" earlier in this section.

With a head, neck, or spinal injury, you may have to control external bleeding. This is why it is important to get the first aid kit. Getting the AED is also important. If the child's condition gets worse, you may need to give CPR until someone with more advanced training arrives and takes over.

Penetrating and Puncturing Injuries

First aid for penetrating and puncturing injuries is different from more common bleeding injuries.

An object such as a knife, nail, or sharp stick can wound a child by penetrating the body or puncturing the skin. If the object is stuck in the body, leave it there until a healthcare provider can treat the injury. Taking it out may cause more bleeding and damage.

Step 1: Prevent

- Supervise children closely whenever they are near common household items that can cause puncture injuries.
- Don't let children play with sharp sticks or toys with sharp points.
- Use the Child and Infant Safety Checklist to help prevent penetrating and puncturing injuries.

Step 2: Protect

- Make sure the scene is safe.
- Get the first aid kit and AED.
- Wear PPE.
- Don't try to pull the object out.

Step 3: Assess

Find the place on the child's body where the object has gone in.

Step 4: Act
Follow these steps to help a child with a penetrating or puncturing injury:

How to Help a Child With a Penetrating or Puncturing Injury
☐ Phone or send someone to phone 9-1-1.
☐ Take steps to stop any bleeding you can see. Do not try to remove the object if it is stuck in the body.
☐ Try to keep the injured child from moving until advanced care arrives and takes over.

Poison Emergencies

A poison is anything that can cause sickness or death if a child swallows it, breathes it, or gets it into the eyes or on the skin. Many medicines, household products, and even some plants can poison children.

Poison Control Hotline

The phone number for the poison control center should be in the first aid kit or clearly posted in the areas where chemicals are used.

Contact your local poison center by phoning the American Association of Poison Control Centers (Poison Control) at

1-800-222-1222

Questions the Poison Control Center Dispatcher May Ask

When you phone the poison control center, they may ask for the following information:

- What is the name of the poison?
- Can you describe it if you can't name it?
- How much poison did the child touch, breathe, or swallow?
- How old is the child?
- How much does the child weigh?
- When did the poisoning happen?
- How is the child feeling or acting now?

Step 1: Prevent

To prevent poisonings, keep items that might be dangerous out of children's reach. Some examples include

- All medicine, including vitamins and supplements
- Mouthwash
- Lamp oil
- Cleaning supplies
- Chemicals

Use the Child and Infant Safety Checklist to help prevent poisoning.

Step 2: Protect

- Take actions to make sure the scene is safe in a poison emergency.
- Get the first aid kit and AED.
- Wear PPE. Whenever possible during CPR, use a mask when giving breaths. This is especially important if the poison is on the child's lips or mouth.

Actions to Take for Scene Safety in a Poison Emergency

☐ Make sure the scene is safe for you and the ill or injured child before you approach.
  • Look for signs that warn you that poisons are nearby (Figure 22).
  • Look for spilled or leaking containers.

☐ If there is a chemical spill or the child is in an unsafe area, try to move the child to an area with fresh air (if you can do so safely).
☐ If the scene seems unsafe, do not approach. Tell everyone to move away.
☐ Stay out of the scene if you see multiple people who may have been poisoned.
☐ Phone or send someone to phone 9-1-1.
☐ Tell the dispatcher the name of the poison if you know it. Some dispatchers may connect you to a poison control center. Give only those antidotes that the poison control center or dispatcher tells you to. The first aid instructions on the poison itself can be helpful but may be incomplete.

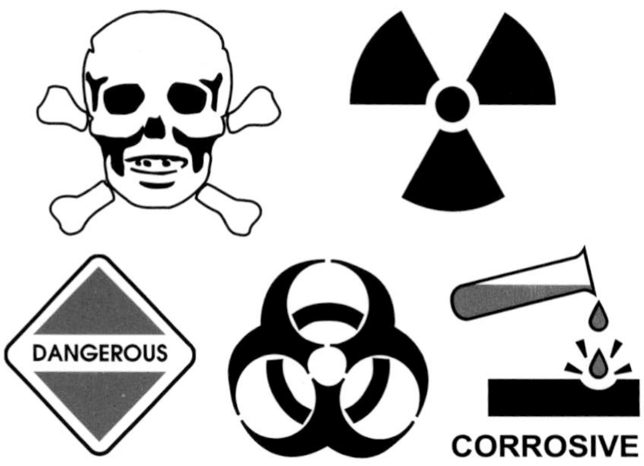

Figure 22. Look for symbols of poisons, such as these.

Safety Data Sheet

Some places have a safety data sheet, or SDS, that describes how a specific chemical or poison can be harmful. It may have first aid recommendations as well.

Step 3: Assess

Suspect that a child has been poisoned if

- You see empty containers that used to hold dangerous contents. Some of these are pill, vitamin, or perfume bottles.
- A child has a chemical smell on his breath or body.
- You suspect the child has eaten parts of a plant.
- You smell something in the room with the child that might be poisonous or dangerous.

Step 4: Act

Follow these steps to help a child who has swallowed a poison:

How to Help a Child Who Has Swallowed Poison
☐ Make sure the scene is safe for you and the ill or injured child before you approach. Follow the steps listed in "Actions to Take for Scene Safety in a Poison Emergency" earlier in this Part.
☐ Move the child away from the poisonous substance. Take the box, bottle, can, or leaf with you for reference when talking to the 9-1-1 dispatcher.
☐ Phone or send someone to phone 9-1-1.
☐ Answer the dispatcher's questions. See "Questions the Poison Control Center Dispatcher May Ask" earlier in this Part.
☐ Tell the dispatcher the name of the poison if you know it. Some dispatchers may connect you to a poison control center.

(continued)

(continued)

How to Help a Child Who Has Swallowed Poison

☐ Give only those antidotes that the poison control center or dispatcher tells you to. The first aid instructions on the poison itself can be helpful but may be incomplete.

☐ Give CPR if the child doesn't respond and is not breathing or only gasping. Use a mask for giving breaths. This is especially important if the poison is on the child's lips or mouth.

Follow these steps to help a child who has poison on the skin or in the eyes:

How to Help a Child With Poison on the Skin or in the Eyes

☐ Make sure the scene is safe for you and the ill or injured child. Follow "Actions to Take for Scene Safety in a Poison Emergency" earlier in this Part.

☐ If you approach the scene, wear PPE.

☐ Move the child from the scene of the poison if you can; help the child move to an area with fresh air.

☐ As quickly and as safely as possible, wash or remove the poison from the child's skin and clothing. Help the child to a faucet, safety shower, or eyewash station.

☐ Remove clothing and jewelry from any part of the body touched by the poison. Use a gloved hand to brush off any dry powder or solid substance from the child's skin (Figure 23A).

☐ Run lots of water over the affected area until someone with more advanced training arrives and takes over.

☐ If an eye is affected, ask the child to blink as much as possible while rinsing the eyes. If only one eye is affected, make sure the eye with the poison in it is lower than the other eye when you rinse (Figure 23B). This will keep the poison from getting into the unaffected eye.

☐ Give CPR if the child doesn't respond and is not breathing or only gasping. Use a mask for giving breaths. This is especially important if the poison is on the child's lips or mouth.

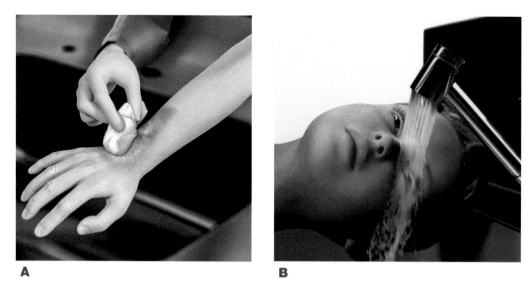

A   B

Figure 23. Remove poisons. **A**, Brush off any dry powder or solid substances. **B**, Rinse the eye.

Seizure

A seizure is abnormal electrical activity in the brain. Most seizures stop within a few minutes. Seizures often are caused by a medical condition called *epilepsy*. In infants and young children, very high fevers can cause seizures. Seizures also can be caused by a head injury, low blood sugar, and heat-related injury. Poisoning and cardiac arrest are other causes.

Signs of a Seizure

Signs of a seizure may differ. Some children who are having a seizure may

- Lose muscle control
- Have jerking movement of the arms, legs, and sometimes other parts of the body
- Fall to the ground
- Lose bowel or bladder control
- Stop responding

However, not all seizures look like this. Other children might become unresponsive. Some might just have a glassy-eyed stare.

During the seizure, a child may bite her tongue, cheek, or mouth. You can give first aid for that injury after the seizure is over. After a seizure, it isn't unusual for the child to be slow to respond and confused. The child may even fall asleep.

Step 1: Prevent

A child's First Aid Action Plan for seizures may list possible triggers to avoid. Sometimes you can't prevent a seizure, but you can prepare for one.

Some children wet or soil their pants during a seizure. Some things you can do to protect a child's privacy and prevent discomfort are

- Cover the child's pants with a blanket after the seizure.
- Have a clean pair of pants for her to change into.

Step 2: Protect

- Make sure the scene is safe. The most important first aid action for a child having a seizure is to protect the child from injury. You may need to move toys and furniture out of the way.
- Get the first aid kit.
- Wear PPE.
- Don't put anything in the child's mouth.

Important: There are many myths about what to do when someone has a seizure. Some tell you to do things that can hurt the child who's having a seizure. (For example, putting a wooden spoon in the mouth can block breathing.) The correct information for how to help a child who is having a seizure is discussed in this workbook and during the course.

Step 3: Assess

Look for signs of seizure listed in this workbook. It is helpful for you to note the time the seizure begins and ends. Observe what happens during and after the seizure. You might need to give this information to the child's caregiver or healthcare provider.

Step 4: Act

Follow these steps to help a child during a seizure:

How to Help a Child During a Seizure
☐ Move furniture or other objects out of the way.
☐ Remove any loose blankets around the child.
☐ Place a small pad or towel under the child's head.

☐ Phone or send someone to phone 9-1-1 if
  • This is the child's first seizure
  • You are unsure whether the child has had a seizure before
  • The First Aid Action Plan for this child says to phone 9-1-1
  • There is more than 1 seizure in a row or seizures do not stop
  • The child is having difficulty breathing because of vomiting or fluids in the mouth
  • The child becomes unresponsive and is not breathing (also start CPR immediately)

Follow these steps to help a child after a seizure:

How to Help a Child After a Seizure

☐ Quickly check to see if the child is responsive and breathing.

☐ Stay with the child until someone with more advanced training arrives and takes over.
  • If the child is having trouble breathing because of vomiting or fluids in her mouth, roll the child onto her side.
  • Give CPR if the child doesn't respond and is not breathing or only gasping.

Mouth and Cheek Injuries

A mouth injury can be serious if blood or broken teeth block the airway. This can cause breathing problems.

Bleeding from the mouth can usually be stopped with pressure.

Step 1: Prevent

Not all mouth and cheek injuries can be prevented. Create a safe environment by proper supervision. Use the Child and Infant Safety Checklist to help prevent injuries.

Step 2: Protect

■ Make sure the scene is safe.
■ Get the first aid kit.
■ Wear PPE.
■ Watch for trouble breathing. Sometimes bleeding in the mouth can block the airway.

Step 3: Assess

Locate the source of the bleeding. The injured area may be inside or outside of the mouth.

Step 4: Act

Follow these steps to help a child with a mouth injury:

How to Help a Child Who Is Bleeding From the Mouth

☐ If bleeding is coming from the tongue, lip, or cheek and you can reach it easily, apply pressure with gauze or a clean cloth (Figure 24).

☐ Phone or send someone to phone 9-1-1 if
  • You can't stop the bleeding
  • The child is having trouble breathing

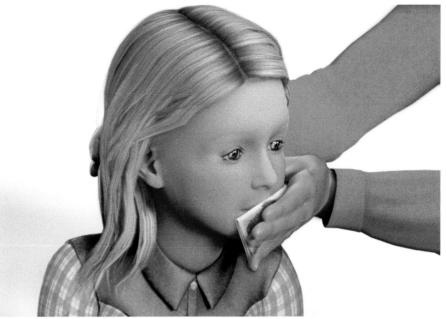

Figure 24. If the bleeding is from the tongue, lip, or cheek, press the bleeding area with sterile gauze or a clean cloth.

Tooth Injuries

Children with a mouth injury may have broken, loose, or knocked-out teeth. These teeth can be a choking hazard, especially for young children.

When a child injures a permanent tooth, sometimes the tooth can be saved. To save the tooth, the child needs immediate first aid care and emergency dental care.

Step 1: Prevent

- Take action to prevent falls.
- Make sure children wear appropriate protective equipment, such as mouth guards when playing sports.
- Use the Child and Infant Safety Checklist to help prevent injuries that lead to tooth injuries.

Step 2: Protect

- Make sure the scene is safe.
- Get the first aid kit.
- Wear PPE.
- If the child has knocked out a tooth, give first aid care and then find the tooth. Hold the tooth by the crown, not the root. Care for the tooth as described below.

Step 3: Assess

- Check the child's mouth for any missing teeth, loose teeth, or parts of teeth.
- If the child has lost a baby tooth, a small amount of bleeding is normal.

Step 4: Act

Follow these steps to help a child with an injury to a permanent tooth:

How to Help a Child With a Permanent Tooth Injury
☐ Check the child's mouth for any missing or loose teeth or parts of teeth.
☐ If a tooth is chipped, gently clean the injured area. Contact a dentist.
☐ If a tooth is loose, have the child bite down on a piece of gauze to keep the tooth in place. Contact a dentist.
☐ If a tooth has come out, it may be possible for a dentist to reattach the tooth. When you hold the tooth, hold it by the crown—the top part of the tooth (Figure 25). Do not hold it by the root; that may injure the root.
☐ Apply pressure with gauze to stop any bleeding in the empty tooth socket.
☐ Clean the area where the tooth was located with saline or clean water.
☐ Put the tooth in one of the following: egg white, coconut water, or whole milk.
☐ If none of these is available, store the tooth in the injured child's saliva. To do this, have the child spit into a container. Then put the tooth in the container. Do not have the child hold the tooth in her mouth.
☐ Immediately take the injured child and tooth to a dentist or emergency department.
☐ Phone or send someone to phone 9-1-1 if you can't control the bleeding.

If a baby tooth is knocked out, stop any bleeding with pressure. Then contact a dentist. You don't need to put the tooth in a solution to preserve it.

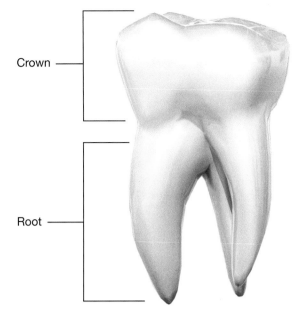

Crown

Root

Figure 25. Hold the tooth by the crown.

Splinters

Splinters are small pieces of wood or metal that stick under the skin. Usually you will not need to phone 9-1-1 for a splinter.

Step 1: Prevent

Supervise children if there is a risk that they may get a splinter, such as on wooden playground equipment.

Step 2: Protect

- Make sure the scene is safe.
- Get the first aid kit.
- Wear PPE.

Step 3: Assess

Find the splinter.

Step 4: Act   Follow these steps to help a child with a splinter:

How to Help a Child With a Splinter

☐ Try to remove the splinter. Keep it dry. If the splinter gets wet, it will be harder to remove it in one piece.
  • If the splinter is small, put sticky tape over the splinter. Then pull the tape off.
  • If tape doesn't pull it out, hold the end of the splinter with clean tweezers. Gently pull it out. (Only pull with the tweezers, without digging).

☐ After you have removed the splinter, clean the child's wound with water and soap if available.

☐ If you can't get a splinter out, leave it in. Clean the area with soap and water. Get medical care if the splinter
  • Is large
  • Is deeply embedded in the skin
  • Is difficult to remove
  • Is in the eye
  • Broke off, possibly leaving part of it in the wound
  • Becomes infected

Illnesses and Injuries: Group B Review Questions

Question	Your Notes
1. What should you do if a child has an injury that needs to be splinted? a. Place a plastic bag filled with warm water on the area to reduce swelling. b. Apply a splint only after an x-ray confirms that the bone is broken. c. Ideally, place the splint so that it supports the joints above and below the injury. d. Straighten the injured body part before using a splint.	

(continued)

Question	Your Notes
2. What should you do when a child gets a small burn? a. Cool the area with cold, but not ice-cold, water. b. Cover the area with lots of cold cream and butter. c. Put the child in a bathtub filled with ice. d. Run warm water on the burn until it doesn't hurt.	
3. Which of the following is true of electrical injuries? a. Electrical injuries have no effect on the heart. b. Electrical injuries never cause injury inside the body. c. High-voltage electricity can travel through everything that touches the power line or source. d. All electrical injuries should be treated with ice.	
4. What should you do if you suspect that a child has a fever? a. Allow the child to play with other children. b. Check his temperature. c. Put ice packs on him. d. Cover him with a blanket.	
5. What is the most important thing to do for a child with a suspected head, neck, or spinal injury? a. Have him sit up. b. Help him walk around. c. Do not twist or turn the head or neck. d. Give him a sports drink.	

(continued)

(continued)

Question	Your Notes
6. If a child has a penetrating injury, you should remove it as quickly as possible. True False	

7. What should you do if a child has a seizure?
 	
  a. Protect the child by moving furniture or other objects out of the way.
 	
  b. Put a spoon in his mouth so he won't bite his tongue.
 	
  c. Pin down his arms and legs so he will not injure them or scare other children.
 	
  d. Turn the child over so he is facedown.	

8. What should you do if a child has a permanent tooth knocked out?
 	
  a. Always hold the tooth by the crown.
 	
  b. Store the tooth in egg white, whole milk, or coconut water.
 	
  c. Immediately take the child and tooth to a dentist or emergency department.
 	
  d. All of the above	

9. What should a child with a nosebleed do?
 	
  a. Lie flat on the ground, facedown
 	
  b. Lean backward as you apply pressure on the soft part of the nose
 	
  c. Blow his nose and then hold an icepack on the back of his neck
 	
  d. Lean forward as you apply pressure on the soft part of the nose	

Answers: 1. c, 2. a, 3. c, 4. b, 5. c, 6. False, 7. a, 8. d, 9. d

Part 4: Preventing Illness and Injury

Injuries are the leading cause of death in children. According to the Centers for Disease Control and Prevention, nearly 9 million children are seen in emergency departments for injuries each year. More than 9000 children die from their injuries annually.

You can help prevent illness and injury to children. Look for possible dangers. Take simple actions to keep children safe. Go to **www.cdc.gov/safechild** for more information.

Topics Covered

Topics covered in this part are

- Car safety and prevention
- Indoor safety and prevention
- Outdoor safety and prevention

For more ways to improve safety and prevent injury, see the Child and Infant Safety Checklist.

Car Safety and Prevention

Injuries from motor vehicle crashes are a leading cause of death in children in the United States. Many of these deaths can be prevented by use of properly installed car seats, booster seats, or seat belts.

Car Seats

Car seats help prevent injuries during car crashes. If appropriate, a car seat should be used every time the child is in a vehicle.

The car seat should

- **Fit the child.** Select a car seat based on the child's age, height, and weight.
- **Be installed correctly.** It should not move more than 1 inch side to side or back to front. Local child car seat inspection stations are available to inspect the car seat. Technicians will make sure it is installed correctly. They will teach you how to install it. In most cases, this service is free. Go to **www.safercar.gov** for more information and to find a location near you.
- **Be used correctly.** Straps should fit snugly. Fasten them securely.

- **Be used each time.** Children should be in a car seat each time they ride in a car. Keep the child in the car seat as long as recommended. Know the height and weight requirements for child safety seat use in your state.

See the Child and Infant Safety Checklist for more information on car seats, booster seats, and seat belts.

Safety in and Around Cars

To help prevent injuries and be safe in the car, remember the following:

- Everyone should wear seat belts.
- All children under 13 years of age should ride in the back seat.
- Never leave a child alone in the car.
- Teach children how to cross streets safely.
- Children should hold hands with or be carried by an adult in parking lots or other places where cars are moving and drivers might not see a child walking.
- Children should cross streets at crosswalks. Teach them street-crossing safety.

For a more complete checklist of things you can do to improve car safety, see the Child and Infant Safety Checklist.

Indoor Safety and Prevention

There are many things that you can do to help keep children safe indoors. Below are some actions to take to prevent poisoning and reduce the risk of sudden infant death syndrome (SIDS).

See the Child and Infant Safety Checklist for other important actions to take. Some of these are preventing falls, burns, and fire injury.

Prevent Poisoning

Some basic actions to prevent injury from poisoning are to

- Keep children away from things that can hurt them. Some of these are medicine, cleaning products, and lamp oil.
- Install smoke and carbon monoxide detectors. Keep working batteries in them.
- Post the poison control center number (1-800-222-1222) near a phone. Add this number to your contacts list in your cell phone.

In a poisoning emergency, phone or send someone to phone 9-1-1. The dispatcher can send help right away if needed and connect you to the poison control center.

Reduce the Risk of SIDS

SIDS is the sudden death of an infant younger than 1 year old that is not explained by other causes.

In the United States, SIDS is a leading cause of death among infants 1 to 12 months old. Although deaths from SIDS have decreased since 1990, rates for some ethnic groups are still high.

To help reduce the risk of SIDS, do the following:

- Put the infant to sleep on her back.
- Make sure the bed has only a mattress, a bottom sheet, and the infant. This means no bumper pads, extra blankets, or stuffed toys.
- Put the infant to sleep in her own bed. Infants should not sleep in the parents' bed. Also, infants can suffocate when they sleep with another child, including a sibling.

Other Actions for Indoor Safety

Here are some other actions for improving indoor safety:

- Install window guards to keep windows from opening completely.
- Put toddler gates at the top and bottom of stairs.
- Supervise children to prevent falls.
- Watch children near water. Infants and young children can drown in bathtubs and toilets.
- Never shake or play roughly with an infant. Shaking or tossing an infant in the air while playing can cause serious injury.

Outdoor Safety and Prevention

There are many things that you can do to help keep children safe outdoors. Below are some actions to take for sports safety and water safety.

See the Child and Infant Safety Checklist for other important actions to take. An example is how to keep children safe when using bikes and skateboards.

Sports Safety

Many childhood injuries happen on the playground. Others occur while children are playing organized sports. Do the following to help keep children safe during play:

- Remove any broken glass or trash from playground areas.
- Have children wear closed-toe shoes.
- Protect children from sunburn.
- In very hot or cold weather, protect children from heat- or cold-related injuries.

- Before a child starts to play a new organized sport, the parents or caregivers should check with a healthcare provider. It is important to identify any health issues that might put the child at risk for illness or injury.
- Children should wear appropriate safety equipment, such as mouth guards and helmets.

Water Safety

Infants and young children can drown in lakes and pools. Drowning can occur in only a few inches of water. Do the following to help reduce the risk of drowning:

- Never leave a child alone around any water.
- An adult must always supervise children while they swim. Never allow a child to swim alone.
- Ensure that home swimming pools have fences. Fences should be 5 feet high on all sides. They should have self-closing, self-latching gates. This includes a gate between the home and the pool.
- Children should wear life jackets in boats and at other times as needed.

Other Actions for Outdoor Safety

Here are some other actions for improving outdoor safety:

- Teach children how to handle and care for a pet.
- Teach children how to behave around dogs, such as
  - Avoiding unfamiliar dogs
  - Asking the owner first before approaching or petting
- Use insect repellent that is approved for use on children.
- Keep children from bothering insects.
- If a child has a known insect allergy, keep her epinephrine pen available whenever the child plays outside.

Child and Infant Safety Checklist

Millions of children are seen for injuries each year in US emergency departments. Injuries are the leading cause of death among children.

Safety checklists can help you identify risks for injury at home, in the car, at childcare facilities, at schools, and on playgrounds. Safety checklists also tell you what to do to reduce risk. But these only reduce risk. There is no such thing as a risk-free environment. That's why it's important to learn first aid.

Action	I follow this safety precaution (✓ = Yes)	Purchase of safety item is required (✓ = Yes)
Car Safety: Car Seats and Seat Belts		
Birth to 12 months A child younger than 1 year old should always ride in a rear-facing car seat. There are different types of rear-facing car seats: • Infant-only seats can only be used rear facing. • Convertible and 3-in-1 car seats typically have higher height and weight limits for the rear-facing position. These allow you to use a rear-facing seat for a longer period of time.		
1 to 4 years Keep a child in a rear-facing car seat as long as recommended. Know the height and weight requirements for child safety seat use in your state. Once the child outgrows the rear-facing car seat, the child is ready to travel in a forward-facing car seat with a harness. The car seat should be placed in the back seat of the automobile.		
4 to 6 years Keep a child in a forward-facing car seat with a harness until he reaches the maximum height or weight limit. Once the child outgrows the forward-facing car seat with a harness, it's time to travel in a booster seat. The booster seat should still be in the back seat.		
6 to 12 years Keep a child in a booster seat until she is big enough to fit in a seat belt properly. For a seat belt to fit properly, the lap belt must lie snugly across the upper thighs, not the stomach. The shoulder belt should lie snugly across the shoulder and chest. It should not cross the neck or face. Remember: The child should still ride in the back seat because it's safer there.		
13 years and older A seat belt should lie across the upper thighs and be snug across the shoulder and chest to restrain the child safely in a crash. It should not rest on the stomach area or across the neck.		
Car Safety: Preventing Injury		
1. Everyone who rides in a car should wear a seat belt.		

(continued)

(continued)

Action	I follow this safety precaution (✓ = Yes)	Purchase of safety item is required (✓ = Yes)
2. All children under 13 years of age should ride in the back seat.		
3. Everyone should keep his or her arms and legs inside the car.		
4. Never leave children alone in or around cars, even for a minute.		
5. Make sure all child passengers have left the vehicle after it is parked.		
6. Take action to make sure you never leave a child in the car. • Put something you'll need, like your cell phone, handbag, employee ID, or briefcase, on the floorboard in the back seat. This will cause you to always look in the back seat before locking the car. • Keep a large stuffed animal in the child's car seat when the child isn't sitting in it. When the child is placed in the seat, put the stuffed animal in the front passenger seat. This will remind you that anytime the stuffed animal is up front, the child is in the back seat in a child safety seat. • Alert your child's day care center or babysitter that you will always phone if your child is not going to be there as scheduled.		
7. Keep vehicles locked at all times, even in the garage or driveway. Always set your parking brake.		
8. Do not leave keys and remote openers within reach of children.		
9. Children should cross streets at cross walks. Teach them street-crossing safety.		
10. Children should hold hands with or be carried by an adult in a parking lot or other places where cars are moving and drivers might not see a child walking.		
Preparation for First Aid Emergencies		
11. Make sure emergency phone numbers are easy to find. Place a sticker or card with these numbers near or on a landline phone; program the numbers into your cell phone. Important numbers include police, fire department, poison control center, hospital emergency services, and healthcare providers. Also include your address and phone number.		
12. Make sure that the building number can be seen from the street. This is so that EMS providers can find it without delay.		

(continued)

(continued)

Action	I follow this safety precaution (✓ = Yes)	Purchase of safety item is required (✓ = Yes)
13. Maintain a fully stocked first aid kit. Know where it is located.		
14. Schools and childcare facilities should have a health record and written First Aid Action Plan for each child with a medical condition.		
Kitchen Safety: Preventing Burns and Other Injury		
15. To reduce the risk of burns • Keep hot liquids, foods, and cooking utensils out of a child's reach. • Place hot liquids and food away from the edge of the table. • Cook on back burners when possible. Turn pot handles toward the center of the stove (away from the front and edges of the stove). • Avoid using tablecloths and placemats that can be pulled, spilling hot liquids or food. • Keep high chairs and stools away from the stove. • Do not keep snacks near the stove. • Do not hold a child or infant while cooking or carrying hot foods or liquids.		
16. Keep knives and other sharp objects out of a child's reach.		
Bathroom Safety: Preventing Injury		
17. Bathe children in no more than 1 or 2 inches of water. Stay with young children and infants throughout bath time. Do not leave small infants or toddlers in the bathtub in the care of young siblings.		
18. Use skidproof mats or stickers in the bathtub. Put a cushioned cover over faucets.		
19. Adjust the maximum temperature of the water heater to 120 degrees Fahrenheit (48.9 degrees Celsius) or below. Test the temperature with a thermometer.		
20. Keep electrical appliances out of the bathroom or unplugged. Keep them away from water and out of a child's reach. This includes radios, hair dryers, and space heaters.		

(continued)

(continued)

Action	I follow this safety precaution (✓ = Yes)	Purchase of safety item is required (✓ = Yes)
Indoor Safety: Preventing Fire Injury		
21. Install smoke detectors in the hallway outside areas where children sleep or nap. Install them on each floor at the head of stairs. Test the alarm each month. Replace batteries once a year. (A good reminder is to replace batteries in the fall when the time changes from daylight saving time.)		
22. Install carbon monoxide detectors. Test them each month.		
23. Make sure that there is an emergency exit from the home, childcare center, classroom, or other area where children are likely to be present. Two exits are preferred. Make sure nothing is blocking the exit(s).		
24. Develop and practice a fire escape plan.		
25. Make sure that a working fire extinguisher is available. This is especially important in areas that have the greatest risk of fire. Some of these areas are the kitchen, furnace room, and near the fireplace.		
26. Make sure that all space heaters are safety approved and in safe operating condition. Place heaters out of a child's reach. They should be at least 3 feet from curtains, papers, and furniture. Heaters should have protective covers.		
27. Make sure all wood-burning stoves and fireplaces are inspected yearly and vented properly. Place stoves out of a child's reach.		
28. Make sure that electrical cords are not frayed or overloaded. Place out of a child's reach.		
29. Keep matches and lighters up high, out of children's sight and reach.		
30. Supervise children if a live candle is in the room. Blow out all candles when you leave the room or go to bed. Avoid the use of candles in the bedroom and other areas where people may fall asleep.		
31. Have flashlights and battery-powered lighting to use during a power outage.		

(continued)

Action	I follow this safety precaution (✓ = Yes)	Purchase of safety item is required (✓ = Yes)
Indoor Safety: Preventing Electrical Injury		
32. Install "shock stops" (plastic outlet plugs) or outlet covers on all electrical outlets.		
33. Make sure cords are not frayed or cracked. Keep cords out of reach of children.		
34. Make sure plugs fit properly into the outlets.		
Indoor Safety: Preventing Falls		
35. Always keep one hand on an infant sitting or lying on a high surface, such as a changing table. Never leave an infant alone on a changing table, couch, bed, or other furniture.		
36. If the infant is in a carrier, place it on the floor rather than on a table, sofa, or bed.		
37. Keep halls and stairs lighted to prevent falls.		
38. Put toddler gates at the top and bottom of stairs. (Do not use accordion-type gates with wide spaces at the top. The child's head could become trapped in such a gate. The child could strangle.)		
39. Infants and children should use stationary activity centers. Avoid infant walkers because they can lead to injuries.		
40. Install window guards to keep windows from opening completely.		
Indoor Safety: Preventing SIDS		
41. Place healthy full-term infants on their backs on a firm mattress to sleep.		
42. Make sure the crib is safe: • The crib mattress should fit snugly, with no more than 2 fingers' width between the mattress and crib railing. • The distance between crib slats should be less than $2\frac{3}{8}$ inches (so the infant's head won't be caught). • Keep all loose blankets, toys, and other items out of the bed. • Keep hanging crib toys out of reach.		
43. Use a crib in good repair. Avoid portable bed rails.		

(continued)

Action	I follow this safety precaution (✓ = Yes)	Purchase of safety item is required (✓ = Yes)
44. Check to see if the crib or mattress has been recalled.		
45. Infants need their own infant beds. The American Academy of Pediatrics does not recommend any bed-sharing arrangements as safe.		
Indoor Safety: Preventing Poisoning		
46. Store medicines and vitamins in child-resistant containers out of a child's reach. Lock drawers and cabinets.		
47. Store cleaning products out of a child's sight and reach. • Store and label all household poisons in their original containers in high, locked cabinets (not under sinks). • Do not store chemicals or poisons in soda bottles. • Store cleaning products away from food.		
48. Install safety latches or locks on cabinets that are within a child's reach and contain possible dangerous items.		
49. Keep purses that contain dangerous items out of a child's reach. Some of these items are vitamins, medicines, cigarettes, and matches. Others are jewelry and calculators. These may have easy-to-swallow button batteries.		
50. Install a lock or hook-and-eye latch on the door to the basement or garage to keep children from entering those areas. Put a lock at the top of the doorframe.		
51. Keep plants that may be harmful out of a child's reach. (Many plants are poisonous. Check with your poison control center.)		
Indoor Safety: Other Prevention Actions		
52. Tie up blind and window curtain cords.		
Preventing Choking		
53. Keep all small items (including food items) that can choke a child out of reach. Test toys for size with a toilet paper roll. If the toy can fit inside the roll, it can choke a child.		

(continued)

(continued)

Action	I follow this safety precaution (✓ = Yes)	Purchase of safety item is required (✓ = Yes)
Toy Safety		
54. Make sure that toy chests have lightweight lids, no lids, or safe-closing hinges.		
55. Follow age recommendations on toy labels.		
Outdoor Safety: Playground		
56. Make sure playground equipment is assembled and anchored correctly according to the manufacturer's instructions. The playground should have a level, cushioned surface, such as sand or wood chips.		
57. Remove any broken glass or trash from playground areas.		
58. Protect children from heat- or cold-related injuries in very hot or cold weather.		
Outdoor Safety: Bikes, Skateboards, Fireworks		
59. Make sure your child knows the rules of safe bicycling: • Wear a protective helmet. • Use the correct-size bicycle. • Ride on the right side of the road (with traffic). • Use hand signals. • Wear bright or reflective clothing. • Never bicycle in the dark or fog. • Young children riding alone should only bike on sidewalks or paths.		
60. Make sure your child is properly protected while roller skating or skateboarding: • Wear a helmet and protective pads on the knees and elbows. • Skate only in rinks or parks that are free of traffic.		
61. Do not allow children to play with fireworks.		
Outdoor Safety: Sports		
62. Make sure your child is properly protected while participating in contact sports: • Children should have proper instruction and adult supervision. • Children should wear appropriate safety equipment, such as mouth guards and helmets.		

(continued)

Action	I follow this safety precaution (✓ = Yes)	Purchase of safety item is required (✓ = Yes)
63. Before a child starts to play a new organized sport, the parents or caregivers should check with a healthcare provider to • Ensure that the child is healthy enough to play the sport • Identify any health issues that might put the child at risk for illness or injury		

Outdoor Safety: Preventing Bites and Stings

Action	I follow this safety precaution (✓ = Yes)	Purchase of safety item is required (✓ = Yes)
64. To reduce the risk of animal bites, teach children the following: • How to handle and care for a pet • To avoid unfamiliar animals • To approach dogs calmly and slowly • To check with the owner first before approaching or petting		
65. To reduce the risk of insect bites and stings, do the following: • Keep children from bothering insects. • Use insect repellent that is approved for use on children. • If you know a child has a severe allergy to an insect bite or bee sting, keep his epinephrine pen close by at all times, especially when the child is outdoors. • Have children wear light-colored clothing that covers the arms and legs when walking or playing in areas where insects are likely to be. • Keep flowering plants and gardens away from areas where children play. • Put outdoor toys away so spiders and insects can't hide inside them.		

Outdoor Safety: Preventing Drowning

Action	I follow this safety precaution (✓ = Yes)	Purchase of safety item is required (✓ = Yes)
66. An adult must always supervise children while they swim. Never allow a child to swim alone.		
67. Closely watch children around any body of water.		
68. Children should wear life jackets in boats and at other times as needed.		
69. Pools and nearby properties should be protected from use by unsupervised children.		

(continued)

(continued)

Action	I follow this safety precaution (✓ = Yes)	Purchase of safety item is required (✓ = Yes)
70. Empty and turn over wading pools as soon as children are done using them.		
71. Do not leave a child alone around any water. A small child or an infant can drown if she falls in a bucket, toilet, or other container filled with water.		
72. If you have a home swimming pool, make sure of the following: • The pool is totally enclosed with fencing. • Fencing is at least 5 feet high. • All gates are self-closing and self-latching. • There is no direct access (without passing through a locked gate) from the home into the pool area.		
73. All adults and older children should learn CPR.		
Outdoor Safety: Preventing Sunburn		
74. Protect children from sunburns: • Keep infants younger than 6 months old out of direct sunlight. • For children older than 6 months, use sunscreen made for children. • Put sunscreen on children 30 minutes before they go outside. • Choose a water-resistant or waterproof sunscreen that blocks both UVA and UVB rays and has an SPF of at least 15. • Reapply waterproof sunscreen every 2 hours, especially if children are playing in the water. • Try to stay out of the sun between 10 AM and 4 PM.		
Firearms: Preventing Firearm Injuries		
75. If firearms are stored in the home, keep them locked. They should be out of a child's sight and reach. Lock and unload each gun before storing it. Store ammunition separate from the firearms.		

The following sources were used in compiling the checklist:

- National Highway Traffic Safety Administration
- Centers for Disease Control and Prevention
- American Academy of Pediatrics
- Safe Kids USA
- KidsAndCars.org
- National Institutes of Health Medline Plus (Gun Safety)
- National Fire Protection Association

Life Is Why

Education Is Why

Heart disease is the No. 1 cause of death in the world—with more than 17 million deaths per year. That's why the AHA is continually transforming our training solutions as science evolves and driving awareness of how everyone can help save a life.

Preventing Illness and Injury: Review Questions

Question	Your Notes
1. To help protect a child from burns, you should a. Keep hot appliances, like irons or curling irons, out of children's reach. b. Keep children away from hot liquids, such as a cup of coffee. c. Cook on the back burners, and keep children away from the stove. d. All of the above	
2. Which of the following reduces the risk of SIDS? a. Putting the infant to sleep on her back b. Putting the infant to sleep on her stomach c. Ensuring that the infant has a First Aid Action Plan d. Ensuring that the infant's car seat is installed correctly	

(continued)

(continued)

Question	Your Notes

3. A correctly installed car seat will not shift more than _____ side to side or back to front.
 	
  a. 1 inch
 	
  b. 1.5 inches
 	
  c. 2 inches
 	
  d. 2.5 inches	

4. In a poisoning emergency, whom should you call first?
 	
  a. An urgent care center
 	
  b. The poison control center
 	
  c. 9-1-1
 	
  d. The child's parent or caregiver	

5. Before a child starts playing an organized sport, the parent or caregiver should
 	
  a. Have his abilities assessed to see if he will be good at the sport
 	
  b. Do nothing—just show up on the first day, ready to play
 	
  c. Check with the child's healthcare provider to identify any illness or injury that might put the child at risk
 	
  d. Wait until the child has played the sport for several weeks to see if any problems develop	

(continued)

Question	Your Notes

6. If a child has a known allergy to bee stings, you should
 	
  a. Not allow the child to participate in outdoor activities
 	
  b. Make sure that the child's epinephrine pen is available at all times
 	
  c. Keep the child inside except during the winter
 	
  d. Call the parent or caregiver if the child gets stung before you do anything else	

7. Which of the following can cause a poisoning emergency?
 	
  a. A button battery
 	
  b. A dishwasher tablet
 	
  c. Blood pressure pills from grandmother's purse
 	
  d. All of the above	

Answers: 1. d, 2. a, 3. a, 4. c, 5. c, 6. b, 7. d

Part 5: First Aid Resources

Topics Covered

Topics covered in this part are

- Sample first aid kit
- Sample First Aid Action Plan
- How children act and tips for interacting with them
- Child abuse and neglect
- Preventing the spread of contagious diseases

Sample First Aid Kit

Below is a sample list of contents for a first aid kit. This kit follows the standard of the Occupational Safety and Health Administration (OSHA). Different workplaces may have different requirements. The American National Standards Institute (ANSI) and the International Safety Equipment Association (ISEA) also have a standard for contents of first aid kits, available at **ansi.org**.

The contents listed below are enough for small workplaces with about 2 or 3 employees. Larger workplaces need more first aid kits or extra supplies.

1. Gauze pads (at least 4 × 4 inches)
2. Two large gauze pads (at least 8 × 10 inches)
3. Box of adhesive bandages
4. One package of gauze roller bandage, at least 2 inches wide
5. Two triangular bandages
6. Wound cleaning agent, such as sealed, moistened towelettes
7. Scissors
8. At least 1 blanket
9. Tweezers
10. Adhesive tape
11. Latex gloves
12. Resuscitation equipment, such as a pocket mask
13. Two elastic wraps
14. Splint
15. Directions for requesting emergency assistance (including list of important local emergency telephone numbers, such as police, fire department, EMS, and poison control center*)
16. Heartsaver First Aid Quick Reference Guide*

*Items marked with an asterisk are in addition to those listed in the OSHA 1910.266 App A standard.

This is a sample only. The actions listed are not for use for an actual child. Always follow instructions from the child's caregiver or physician.

Seizure First Aid Action Plan for
Jimmy Childs

Date of Birth: June 3, 2009
Parents: John and Mary Childs
Parents' Contact Phone Number: 999-452-5555 or 999-321-4444
Jimmy's Physician (for seizures): Dr. AJ Nest, 999-322-3333

Medical Condition: Seizures

Jimmy Childs has a condition known as *epilepsy*. He may have a seizure that will cause him to no longer respond and to have uncontrolled movements of his arms and legs. These seizures usually last a short time. These seizures may last for a longer time or occur with one followed quickly by another. Jimmy's seizures are usually controlled by his medicines, so seizures are unlikely but possible.

Possible triggers:

Bright, flashing lights may trigger a seizure.

Staff members trained to give medicines:

1. Jean Oro
2. Martha Garcia

Staff members trained in First Aid and CPR AED:

1. Jean Oro
2. Martha Garcia
3. Jan Door
4. Stephen Glass

Actions:

Follow first aid actions for seizures as you have been trained to do.

If a seizure lasts longer than 4 minutes or if Jimmy has one seizure followed soon after by another, follow these actions. Only give medicines if you are one of the staff members trained to do so.

1. Have one staff member phone 9-1-1. Let them know a trained staff member will be giving rectal medicine prescribed by Jimmy's physician.
2. The trained staff member will get Jimmy Childs' medicine from the office cabinet. Have another staff member quickly check the label to verify that it is Jimmy's medicine.
3. If Jimmy is still having a seizure, give 1 dose of diazepam rectal gel using the steps printed on the package. (Protect Jimmy's privacy by using screens or moving his classmates out of sight).
4. As soon as possible, contact John or Mary Childs.
5. A first aid–trained staff member will stay with Jimmy at all times.
6. If John or Mary Childs does not arrive by the time the ambulance is ready to transport Jimmy, instruct the emergency providers to take Jimmy to Oceanview Children's Hospital.

After Jimmy is in the care of emergency providers, write a summary. Include what happened before the seizure and during the seizure. Also include what happened after the medicine was given and after the seizure stopped. Provide a copy of this to John or Mary Childs.

Children who are ill, injured, or afraid often do not act their age in years. Instead, they may act like a younger child. Respond to ill, injured, or frightened children based on their behavior, not their age.

The following table explains the characteristics and interaction tips for children of different ages:

Category	Age	Characteristics	Interaction Tips

Infants	Birth to 1 year	• Infants younger than 4 months old may not be able to hold their heads up
		• Cannot talk
		• Will cry to tell you they are
		  – Hungry
		  – Tired
		  – Wet
		  – Want to be held
		  – Scared
		  – Hurt or in pain
			• Support the head when you lift or carry an infant younger than 4 months old.
			• Use a soft, quiet voice when you talk to an infant.
			• Use gentle motions when you approach an infant.
			• Keep the infant warm but not too hot.

Toddlers	1 to 3 years	• Learning to talk
		• Active, moving around and making noise
		• May bite other children when frustrated
		• A toddler who is not active or is acting differently than usual may be
		  – Ill
		  – Injured
		  – Afraid
		  – Tired
			• Toddlers may not speak well themselves.
			• They often can understand what others say.
			• They may be afraid of adults they do not know.
			• You may need to give extra comfort when a healthcare provider arrives to care for a toddler.

Young children	4 to 10 years	• Developmental stages overlap greatly within this age group • Often pick up on the verbal as well as nonverbal behavior of adults around them • Can understand simple explanations • Fear separation from caregivers and friends	• Stay calm. • Use simple words to tell young children what is happening. Be as truthful as possible. Do not lie to the child.

(continued)

Category	Age	Characteristics	Interaction Tips
Adolescents	11 to 18 years	• Understand almost everything around them • Often act without worrying about consequences of their actions • May take risks, such as experimenting with drugs, drinking alcohol, and driving cars • May worry about – How others view them – Whether an injury will be permanent – Getting into trouble because of an injury • May not share information with a first aid rescuer and especially their own parent or caregiver	• Tell them what you are doing to help them. • Reassure them. • Don't disregard the child's complaints and concerns. Make it clear that you are listening carefully.
Children with special needs	Any age	• Have physical, mental, or emotional needs that require special care	• Work with family members or other caregivers to know how to – Use medical devices or medicines – Discuss things with the child

Child Abuse and Neglect

Children of any age can suffer abuse and neglect. Abuse can be caused by parents, caregivers, or others who have a role in caring for the child.

Child abuse happens in every race, ethnicity, and class. The effects of abuse can last a lifetime.

Common Types of Abuse

There are 4 common types of abuse:

Physical abuse	Use of physical force, such as hitting, kicking, or shaking
Sexual abuse	Engaging a child in sexual acts or exposing a child to other sexual activities
Emotional abuse	Behaviors that harm a child's emotional well-being, such as shaming or name calling
Neglect	Failure to meet a child's basic needs, such as housing, food, or access to medical care

Shaken Baby Syndrome

Shaken baby syndrome is a kind of abuse. It happens when someone forcefully shakes an infant. It can severely injure the baby's eyes, neck, or brain. It can cause death.

Signs of Shaken Baby Syndrome

Suspect shaken baby syndrome if an infant has any of the following signs and you can't figure out why:

- Very sleepy or weak
- Very cranky
- Doesn't eat well
- Vomits for no reason
- Doesn't make sounds or smile
- Doesn't suck or swallow well
- Body gets stiff
- Has difficulty breathing
- Has seizures
- Can't lift her head
- Can't focus her eyes or follow movement

If you suspect an infant has suffered from shaken baby syndrome, phone 9-1-1.

Only suspect shaken baby syndrome if you can't explain why the infant has the sign. Sometimes he may be very cranky because he is ill. Another reason may be he missed his nap.

Recognizing Possible Abuse

Children who have been abused may have marks or bruises. They may show signs of abuse in their behavior. Children usually can't or won't talk about the problem.

Sometimes children will tell someone they trust. Take these conversations seriously and report them.

You may suspect abuse if

- A child behaves in certain ways
- A child has physical signs

Behavior Signs of Possible Abuse

A child who has been abused may behave in certain ways. Suspect abuse if the child

- Shows sudden changes in behavior or school performance
- Has unexplained learning problems (or difficulty concentrating)
- Is always watchful, as though preparing for something bad to happen
- Is overly compliant, passive, withdrawn
- Is very demanding and aggressive
- Comes to school or other activities early, stays late, and does not want to go home
- Is uncomfortable with physical contact
- Has low self-esteem
- Lags in physical, emotional, or intellectual development
- Is of very low weight for the child's age
- Has poor growth

Physical Signs of Possible Abuse

A child who has been abused may have physical signs. Suspect abuse if the injuries do not match the caregiver's explanation, including

- Bruises (especially bruises of differing ages and colors)
- Broken bones
- Burns
- Bleeding, cuts, punctures
- Bites
- Blood in the diaper or underwear
- Trouble walking or sitting
- Untreated dental problems
- Headaches
- Stomachaches
- Poisoning
- Seizures
- Vomiting

To Report Abuse or Get Help

Reporting suspected abuse can help both the child and the family. If the abuse is not reported, the child will continue to be in danger. Sometimes child abuse can result in death.

In many states, anyone who suspects child abuse is required to report it. Phone the National Child Abuse Hotline at 1-800-4-A-CHILD (1-800-422-4453) to report a problem or to get help. All calls to this hotline are anonymous.

The identity of a person who reports child abuse is confidential. It can only be disclosed by court order or to a law enforcement officer involved in the investigation.

It is important to remember that the person who reports suspected abuse is responsible only for reporting the information. It is the role of law enforcement to determine if abuse is present.

To Learn More

To learn more about child abuse, see the following:

Centers for Disease Control and Prevention
www.cdc.gov/violenceprevention

Centers for Disease Control Facebook Page on Violence Prevention
www.facebook.com/VetoViolence

Children's Bureau
www.acf.hhs.gov/programs/cb

Child Welfare Information Gateway
www.childwelfare.gov

FRIENDS National Center for Community-Based Child Abuse Prevention
www.friendsnrc.org

Sources

In addition to the links above, the following sources also were used in compiling the abuse information:

National Center on Shaken Baby Syndrome
http://dontshake.org

About Shaken Baby
www.aboutshakenbaby.com

Maryland and Oregon State Governments
www.maryland.gov
www.oregon.gov

National Institutes of Health
www.nlm.nih.gov/medlineplus/childabuse.html

Mayo Clinic
www.mayoclinic.org

Contagious diseases are a leading cause of illness and death in the United States. Vaccines are available that prevent these diseases. Good handwashing is essential to any disease prevention. Go to the following websites to learn more:

- www.cdc.gov/vaccines
- www.vaccines.gov
- www.cdc.gov/flu/protect/preventing.htm
- www.cdc.gov/vaccinesafety/index.html

Part 6: Pediatric First Aid Skills Summary

Topics Covered

This part is a review of important first aid skills that you will have an opportunity to practice and demonstrate during the course:

- Remove protective gloves
- Find the problem
- Control bleeding by direct pressure and bandaging
- Use an epinephrine pen
- Apply a splint (optional)

Remove Protective Gloves

Here is the correct way to remove protective gloves (Figure 26):

How to Remove Protective Gloves

☐ Grip one glove on the outside near the cuff, and peel it down until it comes off inside out (Figure 26A).

☐ Cup it with your other gloved hand (Figure 26B).

☐ Place 2 fingers of your bare hand inside the cuff of the glove that is still on your other hand (Figure 26C).

☐ Peel that glove off so that it comes off inside out with the first glove inside it (Figure 26D).

☐ If blood or blood-containing material is on the gloves, dispose of the gloves properly.
- Put the gloves in a biohazard waste bag.
- If you do not have a biohazard waste bag, put the gloves in a plastic bag that can be sealed before you dispose of it.

☐ Wash your hands well. You should always wash your hands after removing gloves, just in case some blood or body fluids came in contact with your hands.

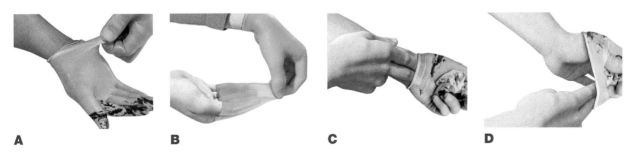

A   **B**   **C**   **D**

Figure 26. Proper removal of protective gloves without touching the outside of the gloves.

Find the Problem

Here are the steps to take to find the problem. They are listed in order of importance, with the most important step listed first.

How to Find the Problem
☐ Make sure the scene is safe.
☐ Check to see if the child responds. Approach the child, tap him, and shout, "Are you OK? Are you OK?"

If the child is *responsive*	If the child is *unresponsive*
☐ Ask what the problem is if the child is old enough to talk.	☐ Shout for help/phone 9-1-1. • Phone or send someone to phone 9-1-1 and get a first aid kit and AED. • If possible, put the phone on speaker mode when you phone 9-1-1.
☐ If the child only moves, moans, or groans, shout for help. Phone or send someone to phone 9-1-1 and get the first aid kit and AED.	☐ Check for breathing. • If the child is not breathing or is only gasping, begin CPR and use an AED. See the "CPR and AED" part later in this workbook. • If the child is breathing, stay with the child until advanced help arrives. • Check for injuries and medical information jewelry.
☐ Check the child's breathing. • If the child is breathing without difficulty and doesn't need immediate first aid, look for any obvious signs of injury, such as bleeding, broken bones, burns, or bites. • Look for any medical information jewelry. This tells you if the child has a serious medical condition.	☐ Stay with the child until someone with more advanced training arrives and takes over.

Control Bleeding by Direct Pressure and Bandaging

Here are the steps to stop bleeding:

☐ Apply dressings from the first aid kit. Put direct pressure on the dressings over the bleeding area. Use the flat part of your fingers or the palm of your hand (Figure 27).

☐ If the bleeding doesn't stop, you'll need to add more dressings and press harder. Do not remove a dressing once it's in place because this could cause the wound to bleed more. Keep pressure on the wound until it stops bleeding.

☐ Once the bleeding has stopped or if you can't keep pressure on the wound, wrap a bandage firmly over the dressings to hold them in place.

☐ For minor cuts and scrapes, wash the area with soap and water once the bleeding has stopped. Then apply a dressing to the wound.

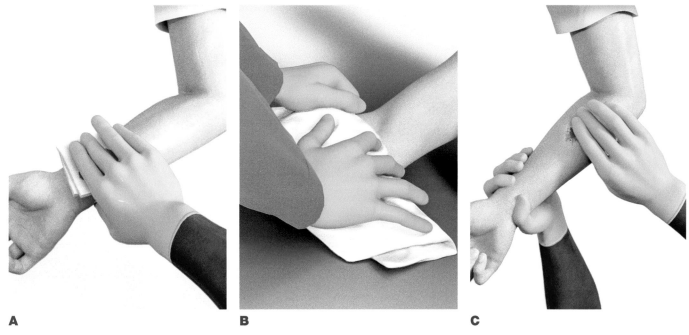

A   B   C

Figure 27. Controlling bleeding. **A**, A dressing can be a gauze pad or pads. **B**, It can be any other clean piece of cloth. **C**, If you do not have a dressing, use your gloved hand.

Use an Epinephrine Pen

Here are the steps to help someone with signs of a severe allergic reaction use his epinephrine pen:

How to Use an Epinephrine Pen

☐ Follow the instructions on the pen. Make sure you are holding the pen in your fist without touching either end because the needle comes out of one end. You may give the injection through clothes or on bare skin.

☐ Take off the safety cap (Figure 28A).

☐ Press the tip of the injector hard against the side of the child's thigh, about halfway between the hip and the knee (Figure 28B).

☐ Hold the pen in place for about 10 seconds.

☐ Pull the pen straight out. Make sure you don't put your fingers over the end that has been pressed against the child's thigh.

☐ Either the child getting the injection or the person giving the injection should rub the injection spot for about 10 seconds.

☐ Note the time of the injection. Give the pen to the emergency providers for proper disposal.

☐ If the child doesn't get better or if advanced care doesn't arrive within 10 minutes
  • Phone or send someone to phone 9-1-1
  • Consider giving a second dose, if one is available

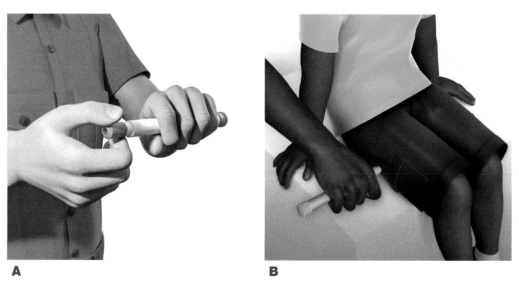

A   B

Figure 28. Using an epinephrine pen. **A**, Take off the safety cap. **B**, Press the tip of the injector hard against the side of the child's thigh, about halfway between the hip and the knee.

Assemble and Use an Inhaler

Here are the steps to assemble and use an inhaler:

How to Assemble and Use an Inhaler

To assemble the inhaler

☐ First, shake the medicine.

☐ Put the medicine canister into the mouthpiece.

☐ Remove the cap from the mouthpiece.

☐ Attach a spacer if there is one available and if you know how.

To help a child use an inhaler, ask him to do the following:

☐ Tilt his head back slightly and breathe out slowly.

☐ Place the inhaler or spacer in his mouth.

☐ Push down on the medicine canister.

☐ Breathe in very deeply and slowly.

☐ Hold his breath for about 10 seconds.

☐ Then breathe out slowly.

Apply a Splint

Here are the steps to apply a splint:

How to Apply a Splint

☐ Find an object that you can use to keep the injured arm or leg from moving.

☐ Rolled-up towels, magazines, and pieces of wood can be used as splints. Splint in a way to reduce pain and limit further injury. The splint should be longer than the injured area. It should support the joints above and below the injury.

☐ After covering any broken skin with a clean or sterile cloth, tie or tape the splint to the injured limb so that it supports the injured area.

☐ Use tape, gauze, or cloth to secure it. It should fit snugly but not cut off circulation.

☐ If you're using a hard splint, like wood, make sure you pad it with something soft, like clothing or a towel.

☐ Keep the limb still until the injured child can be seen by a healthcare provider.

CPR and AED

Although much is being done to prevent death from heart problems, sudden cardiac arrest is still one of the leading causes of death in the United States. About 70% of the arrests that occur outside of the hospital happen at home.

In this part, you will learn skills that will help you to recognize cardiac arrest, get emergency care on the way quickly, and help the person until more advanced care arrives to take over.

Life Is Why

High-Quality CPR Is Why

Early recognition and CPR are crucial for survival from cardiac arrest. By learning high-quality CPR, you'll have the knowledge and skills that may help save a life.

CPR AED Course Objectives

At the end of the CPR AED portion of this course, you will be able to

- Describe how high-quality CPR improves survival
- Explain the concepts of the Chain of Survival
- Recognize when someone needs CPR
- Perform high-quality CPR for an adult
- Describe how to perform CPR with help from others
- Give effective breaths by using mouth-to-mouth or a mask for all age groups
- Demonstrate how to use an AED on an adult
- Perform high-quality CPR for a child
- Demonstrate how to use an AED on a child
- Perform high-quality CPR for an infant
- Describe when and how to help a choking adult or child
- Demonstrate how to help a choking infant

Sudden Cardiac Arrest

Sudden Cardiac Arrest vs Heart Attack

People often use the terms *sudden cardiac arrest* and *heart attack* to mean the same thing—but they are not the same.

Sudden cardiac arrest is a "rhythm" problem. It occurs when the heart malfunctions and stops beating unexpectedly.

A *heart attack* is a "clot" problem. It occurs when a clot blocks blood flow.

Sudden Cardiac Arrest

Sudden cardiac arrest results from an abnormal heart rhythm. This abnormal rhythm causes the heart to quiver so that it can no longer pump blood to the brain, lungs, and other organs.

Within seconds, the person becomes unresponsive and is not breathing or is only gasping. Death occurs within minutes if the person does not receive immediate lifesaving treatment.

Heart Attack

A heart attack occurs when blood flow to part of the heart muscle is blocked by a clot. Typically during a heart attack, the heart continues to pump blood.

A person having a heart attack may have discomfort or pain in the chest. There may be an uncomfortable feeling in one or both arms, the neck, the jaw, or the back between the shoulder blades.

The longer the person with a heart attack goes without treatment, the greater the possible damage to the heart muscle. Occasionally, the damaged heart muscle triggers an abnormal rhythm that can lead to sudden cardiac arrest.

CPR and AED Use for Adults

What You Will Learn

In this section, you will learn when CPR is needed, how to give CPR to an adult, and how to use an AED.

Adult Chain of Survival

The AHA adult Chain of Survival (Figure 29) shows the most important actions needed to treat adults who have cardiac arrests outside of a hospital.

In this part, you will learn about the first 3 links of the chain. The fourth and fifth links are advanced care provided by emergency responders and hospital providers who will take over care.

First link	Immediately recognize the emergency and phone 9-1-1.
Second link	Perform early CPR with an emphasis on chest compressions.
Third link	Use an AED immediately (as soon as it is available).

Remember that seconds count when someone has a cardiac arrest. Wherever you are, take action. The adult Chain of Survival starts with you!

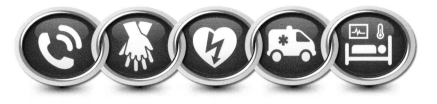

Figure 29. The AHA adult Chain of Survival for cardiac arrests that occur outside of a hospital.

Topics Covered

- Assess and phone 9-1-1
- Perform high-quality CPR
- Use an AED
- Putting it all together: adult high-quality CPR AED summary

Assess and Phone 9-1-1

When you encounter an adult who may have had a cardiac arrest, take the following steps to assess the emergency and get help:

- Make sure the scene is safe.
- Tap and shout (check for responsiveness).
- Shout for help.
- Phone 9-1-1 and get an AED.
- Check for normal breathing.

Depending on the particular circumstance and the resources you have available, you may be able to perform some of these actions at the same time. You might, for example, phone 9-1-1 with your cell phone on speaker mode while checking for breathing.

Make Sure the Scene Is Safe

Before you assess the person, make sure the scene is safe. Look for anything nearby that might hurt you. You can't help if you get hurt too.

Some places that may be unsafe are

- A busy street or parking lot
- An area where power lines are down
- A room with poisonous fumes

As you give care, be aware if anything changes and makes it unsafe for you or the person needing help.

Tap and Shout (Check for Responsiveness)

Tap and shout to check if the person is responsive or unresponsive (Figure 30). Lean over the person or kneel at his side. Tap his shoulders and ask if he is OK.

If	Then
The person moves, speaks, blinks, or otherwise reacts when you tap him.	• He is *responsive*. • Ask the person if he needs help.
The person doesn't move, speak, blink, or otherwise react when you tap him.	• He is *unresponsive*. • Shout for help so that if others are nearby, they can help you.

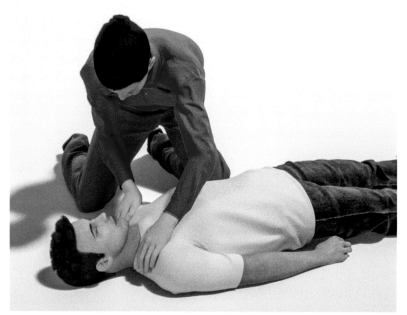

Figure 30. Tap and shout (check for responsiveness).

Shout for Help

In an emergency, the sooner you realize that there's a problem and get additional help, the better it is for the person with a cardiac arrest. When more people are helping, you are able to provide better care to the person.

If the person is unresponsive, shout for help (Figure 31).

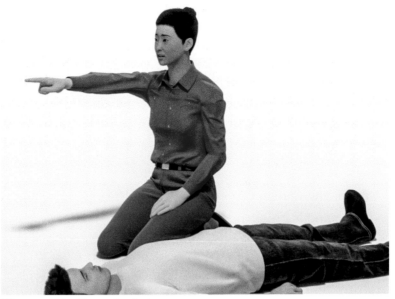

Figure 31. Shout for help.

Phone 9-1-1 and Get an AED

If someone comes to help and a cell phone is available

Ask the person to phone 9-1-1 and get an AED. Say, "You—phone 9-1-1 and get an AED." Ask that the phone be placed on speaker mode so that you can hear the dispatcher's instructions.

If someone comes to help and a cell phone is not available

Ask the person to go phone 9-1-1 and get an AED while you continue providing emergency care.

If you are alone and have a cell phone or nearby phone

If no one comes to help, phone 9-1-1. Put the phone on speaker mode so that you can hear the dispatcher's instructions while you continue providing emergency care. If an AED is needed, you will have to go get it yourself.

If you are alone and don't have a cell phone

Leave the person to go phone 9-1-1 and get an AED. Return and continue providing emergency care.

Follow the Dispatcher's Instructions

Stay on the phone until the 9-1-1 dispatcher tells you to hang up. Answering the dispatcher's questions will not delay the arrival of help.

The dispatcher will ask you about the emergency—where you are and what has happened. Dispatchers can provide instructions that will help you, such as telling you how to provide CPR, use an AED, or give first aid.

That's why it's important to put the phone on speaker mode after phoning 9-1-1 so that the dispatcher and the person providing CPR can speak to each other.

Check for Normal Breathing

If the person is unresponsive, check for normal breathing (Figure 32).

Scan the chest from head to chest repeatedly for at least 5 seconds (but no more than 10 seconds) looking for chest rise and fall. If the person is not breathing normally or is only gasping, he needs CPR. (See "Heartsaver Pediatric First Aid CPR AED Terms and Concepts" for more information on gasping.)

If	Then
The person is unresponsive and is breathing normally.	• This person does not need CPR. • Roll him onto his side (if you don't think he has a neck or back injury). This will help keep the airway clear in the event the person vomits. • Stay with the person until advanced help arrives.
The person is unresponsive and not breathing normally or is only gasping.	• This person needs CPR. • Make sure the person is lying on his back on a firm, flat surface. • Begin CPR.

Remember

Unresponsive
+
No normal breathing
or only gasping

=

Provide CPR

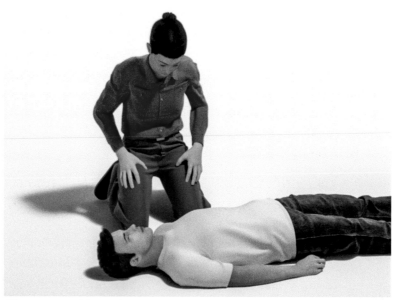

Figure 32. Check for normal breathing.

What to Do If You Are Not Sure

If you think someone needs CPR but you aren't sure, provide CPR because you may save a life. CPR is not likely to cause harm if the person is not in cardiac arrest.

It's better to give CPR to someone who doesn't need it than not to give it to someone who does need it.

Summary

Here is a summary of how to assess the emergency and get help when you encounter an ill or injured adult:

Assess and Phone 9-1-1

☐ Make sure the scene is safe.

☐ Tap and shout (check for responsiveness).
- If the person is *responsive*, ask him if he needs help.
- If the person is *unresponsive*, go to the next step.

☐ Shout for help.

☐ Phone 9-1-1 and get an AED.
- Phone or send someone to phone 9-1-1 and get an AED.
- If you're alone and have a cell phone or a nearby phone, put it on speaker mode and call 9-1-1.

☐ Check for breathing.
- If the person is breathing normally, stay with the person until advanced help arrives.
- If the person is *not* breathing normally or only gasping, begin CPR and use an AED. See "Perform High-Quality CPR."

Perform High-Quality CPR

Learning how to perform high-quality CPR is important. The better the CPR skills are performed, the better the chances of survival.

Life Is Why

Saving Lives Is Why

Sudden cardiac arrest remains a leading cause of death, so the American Heart Association trains millions of people each year to help save lives both in and out of the hospital.

CPR Skills

CPR has 2 main skills:

- Providing compressions
- Giving breaths

You will learn how to perform these skills for an adult in cardiac arrest in this section.

Provide Compressions

A compression is the act of pushing hard and fast on the chest. When you push on the chest, you pump blood to the brain and heart.

To provide high-quality compressions, make sure that you

- Provide compressions that are deep enough
- Provide compressions that are fast enough
- Let the chest come back up to its normal position after each compression
- Try not to interrupt compressions for more than 10 seconds, even when you give breaths

Compression depth is an important part of providing high-quality compressions. You need to push hard enough to pump blood through the body. It's better to push too hard than not hard enough. People are often afraid of causing a person injury by providing compressions, but injury is unlikely.

Compression Technique

Here is how to provide compressions for an adult during CPR (Figure 33):

How to Provide Compressions for an Adult During CPR
☐ Make sure the person is lying on his back on a firm, flat surface.
☐ Quickly move clothes out of the way.
☐ Put the heel of one hand on the center of the chest (over the lower half of the breastbone). Put your other hand on top of the first hand (Figure 33).
☐ Push straight down at least 2 inches.
☐ Push at a rate of 100 to 120 compressions per minute. Count the compressions out loud.
☐ Let the chest come back up to its normal position after each compression.
☐ Try not to interrupt compressions for more than 10 seconds, even when you give breaths.

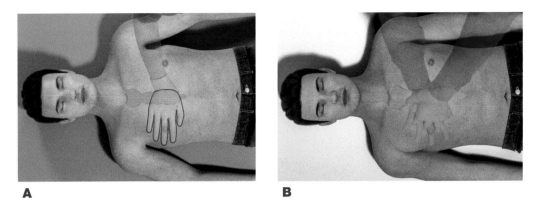

A

B

Figure 33. Compressions. **A,** Put the heel of one hand on the center of the chest (lower half of the breastbone). **B,** Put the other hand on top of the first hand.

Switch Rescuers to Avoid Fatigue

Performing chest compressions correctly is hard work. The more tired you become, the less effective your compressions will be.

If someone else knows CPR, you can take turns providing CPR (Figure 34). Switch rescuers about every 2 minutes, or sooner if you get tired. Move quickly to keep any pauses in compressions as short as possible.

Remind other rescuers to perform high-quality CPR as described in the table labeled "How to Provide Compressions for an Adult During CPR."

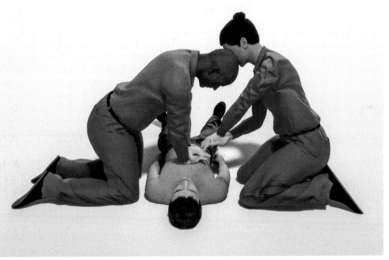

Figure 34. Switch rescuers about every 2 minutes to avoid fatigue.

Give Breaths

The second skill of CPR is giving breaths. After each set of 30 compressions, you will need to give 2 breaths. Breaths may be given with or without a barrier device, such as a pocket mask or face shield.

When you give breaths, the breaths need to make the chest rise visibly. When you can see the chest rise, you know you have delivered an effective breath.

Before giving breaths, open the airway (Figure 35). This lifts the tongue from the back of the throat to make sure your breaths get air into the lungs.

Follow these steps to open the airway:

How to Open the Airway
☐ Put one hand on the forehead and the fingers of your other hand on the bony part of the chin (Figure 35).
☐ Tilt the head back and lift the chin.

Avoid pressing into the soft part of the neck or under the chin because this might block the airway.

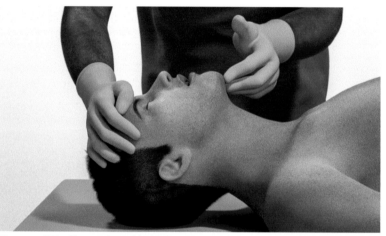

Figure 35. Open the airway by tilting the head back and lifting the chin.

Give Breaths Without a Pocket Mask

If you choose to give someone breaths without a barrier device, it is usually quite safe because there is very little chance that you will catch a disease.

How to Give Breaths Without a Pocket Mask
☐ While holding the airway open, pinch the nose closed with your thumb and forefinger.
☐ Take a normal breath. Cover the person's mouth with your mouth.
☐ Give 2 breaths (blow for 1 second for each) (Figure 36). Watch for the chest to begin to rise as you give each breath.
☐ Try not to interrupt compressions for more than 10 seconds.

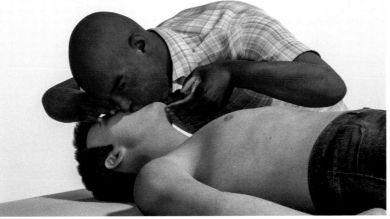

Figure 36. Give breaths.

What to Do If the Chest Doesn't Rise

It takes a little practice to give breaths correctly. If you give someone a breath and the chest doesn't rise, do the following:

- Allow the head to go back to its normal position.
- Open the airway again by tilting the head back and lifting the chin.
- Then, give another breath. Make sure the chest rises.

Minimize Interruptions in Chest Compressions

If you have been unable to give 2 effective breaths in 10 seconds, go back to pushing hard and fast on the chest. Try to give breaths again after every 30 compressions.

Don't interrupt compressions for more than 10 seconds.

Use a Pocket Mask

You may give breaths with or without a barrier device, such as a pocket mask. Barrier devices are made of plastic and fit over the person's mouth and nose (Figure 37). They protect the rescuer from blood, vomit, or disease. Your instructor may discuss other types of barrier devices, like face shields, which can be used when giving breaths.

If you're in the workplace, your employer may provide personal protective equipment, including pocket masks or face shields, for use during CPR.

There are many different kinds of pocket masks as well as different sizes for adults, children, and infants. So, make sure you're using the right size. You may need to put a pocket mask together before you use it.

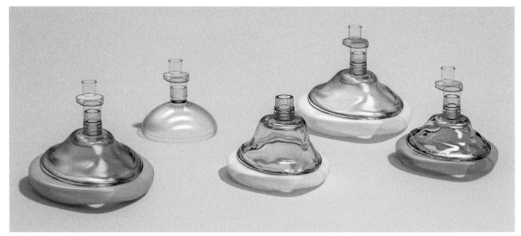

Figure 37. Some people use a pocket mask when giving breaths.

Give Breaths With a Pocket Mask

Follow these steps to give breaths with a pocket mask (Figure 38):

How to Give Breaths With a Pocket Mask

☐ Put the mask over the person's mouth and nose.
- If the mask has a pointed end, put the narrow end of the mask on the bridge of the nose; position the wide end so that it covers the mouth.

☐ Tilt the head and lift the chin while pressing the mask against the person's face. It is important to make an airtight seal between the person's face and the mask while you lift the chin to keep the airway open.

☐ Give 2 breaths (blow for 1 second for each). Watch for the chest to begin to rise as you give each breath.

☐ Try not to interrupt compressions for more than 10 seconds.

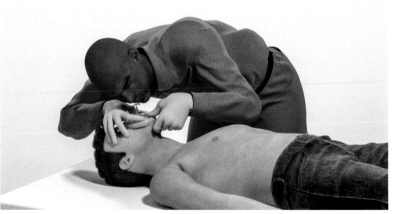

Figure 38. Giving breaths with a pocket mask.

Give Sets of 30 Compressions and 2 Breaths

When providing CPR, give sets of 30 compressions and 2 breaths.

How to Give Sets of Compressions and Breaths to an Adult
☐ Make sure the person is lying on his back on a firm, flat surface.
☐ Quickly move clothes out of the way.

☐ Give 30 chest compressions.
    • Put the heel of one hand on the center of the chest (over the lower half of the breastbone.) Put your other hand on top of the first hand.
    • Push straight down at least 2 inches.
    • Push at a rate of 100 to 120 compressions per minute. Count the compressions out loud.
    • Let the chest come back up to its normal position after each compression.

☐ After 30 compressions, give 2 breaths.
    • Open the airway and give 2 breaths (blow for 1 second for each). Watch for the chest to begin to rise as you give each breath.
    • Try not to interrupt compressions for more than 10 seconds.

Use an AED

CPR combined with using an AED provides the best chance of saving a life. If possible, use an AED every time you provide CPR.

AEDs are safe, accurate, and easy to use. Once you turn on the AED, follow the prompts. The AED will analyze if the person needs a shock and will automatically give one or tell you when to give one.

Turn on the AED

To use an AED, turn it on by either pushing the "on" button or lifting the lid (Figure 39). Once you turn on the AED, you will hear prompts, which will tell you everything you need to do.

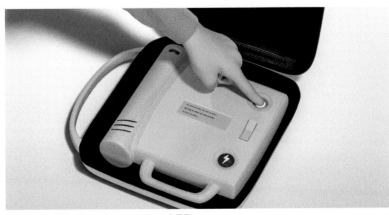

Figure 39. Turning on the AED.

Attach the Pads

AEDs may have adult and child pads. Make sure you use the adult pads for anyone 7 years of age or older. Before you place the pads, quickly scan the person to see if there are any special situations that might require additional steps. See "Special Situations" later in this section.

Peel away the backing from the pads. Following the pictures on the pads, attach them to the person's bare chest (Figure 40).

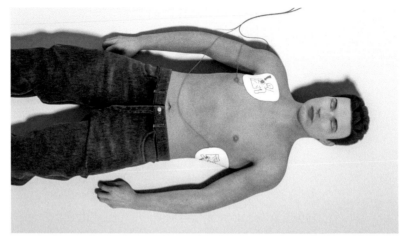

Figure 40. Place pads on an adult by following the pictures on the pads.

Clear the Person If a Shock Is Advised

Let the AED analyze the heart rhythm. If the AED advises a shock, it will tell you to stay clear of the person. If so, then loudly state, "Clear." Make sure that no one is touching the person just before you push the "shock" button (Figure 41).

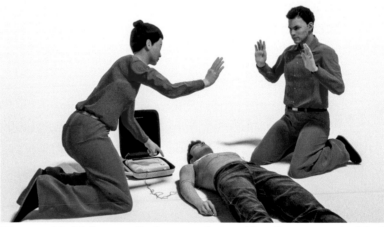

Figure 41. Make sure that no one is touching the person just before you push the "shock" button.

Steps for Using an AED for an Adult

Use the AED as soon as it is available. Here are the steps for using an AED for an adult:

How to Use an AED for an Adult

☐ Turn the AED on and follow the prompts.
  • Turn it on by pushing the "on" button or lifting the lid (Figure 39).
  • Follow the prompts, which will tell you everything you need to do.

☐ Attach the adult pads.
  • Use the adult pads for anyone 8 years of age and older.
  • Peel away the backing from the pads.
  • Following the pictures on the pads, attach them to the person's bare chest (Figure 40).

☐ Let the AED analyze.
  • Loudly state, "Clear," and make sure that no one is touching the person.
  • The AED will analyze the heart rhythm.
  • If a shock is not needed, resume CPR.

☐ Deliver a shock if needed (Figure 41).
  • Loudly state, "Clear," and make sure that no one is touching the person.
  • Push the "shock" button.
  • Immediately resume CPR.

Special Situations

There are some special situations that you may need to consider before placing AED pads. Quickly scan the person to see if he has any of the following *before* applying the pads:

If the person...	Then

Has hair on the chest that may prevent pads from sticking	• Quickly shave the area where you will place the pads by using the razor from the AED carrying case.
	or
	• Remove the hair by using a second set of AED pads (if available).
	  – Apply the pads and press them down firmly.
	  – Rip the pads off forcefully to remove the chest hair.
	  – Reapply a new set of pads to the bare skin.

Is lying in water	• Quickly move the person to a dry area.
Is lying on snow or in a small puddle	• You may use the AED (the chest doesn't have to be completely dry). • If the chest is covered with water or sweat, quickly wipe it before attaching the pads.

(continued)

(continued)

If the person...	Then
Has water on the chest	• Quickly wipe the chest dry before attaching the pads.
Has an implanted defibrillator or pacemaker	• Don't put the AED pad directly over the implanted device. • Follow the normal steps for operating an AED.
Has a medicine patch where you need to place an AED pad	• Don't put the AED pad directly over a medicine patch. • Use protective gloves. • Remove the medicated patch. • Wipe the area clean. • Attach the AED pads.

Continue Providing CPR and Using the AED

As soon as the AED gives the shock, immediately resume chest compressions. Continue to follow the AED prompts, which will guide the rescue.

Provide CPR and use the AED until

- Someone else arrives who can take turns providing CPR with you
- The person begins to move, speak, blink, or otherwise react
- Someone with more advanced training arrives

Putting It All Together: Adult High-Quality CPR AED Summary

Compressions are very important to deliver blood flow and are the core of CPR. Try not to interrupt chest compressions for more than 10 seconds when you give breaths.

Assess and Phone 9-1-1

☐ Make sure the scene is safe.

☐ Tap and shout (check for responsiveness).
- If the person is *responsive*, ask him if he needs help.
- If the person is *unresponsive*, go to the next step.

☐ Shout for help.

☐ Phone 9-1-1 and get an AED.
- Phone or send someone to phone 9-1-1 and get an AED.
- If you're alone and have a cell phone or a nearby phone, put it on speaker mode and call 9-1-1.

(continued)

(continued)

☐ Check for breathing.
  - If the person is breathing normally, stay with the person until advanced help arrives.
  - If the person is *not* breathing normally or only gasping, begin CPR and use an AED. See the next steps.

Provide High-Quality CPR

When providing CPR, you give sets of 30 compressions and 2 breaths.

☐ Make sure the person is lying on his back on a firm, flat surface.

☐ Quickly move clothes out of the way.

☐ Give 30 chest compressions.
  - Put the heel of one hand on the center of the chest (over the lower half of the breastbone). Put your other hand on top of the first hand.
  - Push straight down at least 2 inches.
  - Push at a rate of 100 to 120 compressions per minute. Count the compressions out loud.
  - Let the chest come back up to its normal position after each compression.

☐ After 30 compressions, give 2 breaths.
  - Open the airway and give 2 breaths (blow for 1 second for each). Watch for the chest to begin to rise as you give each breath.
  - Try not to interrupt compressions for more than 10 seconds, even when you give breaths.

☐ Use an AED as soon as it is available.
  - Turn the AED on and follow the prompts.
  - Attach the adult pads.
  - Let the AED analyze.
  - Make sure no one is touching the person, and deliver a shock if advised.

☐ Provide CPR and use the AED until
  - Someone else arrives who can take turns providing CPR with you
  - The person begins to move, speak, blink, or otherwise react
  - Someone with more advanced training arrives and takes over

In the United States, drug overdoses now kill more adults each year than motor vehicle crashes do. Many overdoses are from prescription drugs. Opioids are prescription drugs used for pain relief but are often abused. Common opioids are morphine and hydrocodone. Heroin is an example of an opioid that is illegal in the United States.

Naloxone Reverses Effects of Opioids

Naloxone is a drug that reverses the effects of opioids. It is safe and effective. Emergency responders have used naloxone for many years.

Family members or caregivers of known opioid users may have naloxone close by to use in case of an opioid overdose.

If you know someone who has a prescription for naloxone, you may have to use it. It is important to be familiar with how to use naloxone.

Facts About Naloxone

Here are some facts about naloxone:

How to get it	Naloxone is available by prescription and through substance abuse treatment programs.
How to use it	Naloxone comes in several forms. Common forms are an intranasal spray or autoinjector (similar to an epinephrine pen). Give naloxone by spraying it into the nose or by injecting it into a muscle with an autoinjector.
Who can give it	Naloxone should be given only by someone who has been trained and can identify an opioid overdose.
When to give it	Naloxone is used to reverse the effects of an opioid overdose. It won't work for other types of drug overdoses.

Actions to Help an Adult With an Opioid-Associated Emergency

If you suspect that someone has had an opioid overdose and the person is still responsive, phone 9-1-1 and stay with the person until someone with more advanced training arrives.

If the person becomes unresponsive, follow these steps:

☐ Shout for help.

☐ If someone is nearby, have that person phone 9-1-1 and get the naloxone kit and AED. Use the naloxone as soon as it arrives.

☐ Check for breathing.

☐ If no one is nearby and the person isn't breathing normally or is only gasping, provide CPR. After 5 cycles of CPR, phone 9-1-1 and get the naloxone and AED.

☐ Return to the person and give the naloxone. Check for responsiveness and breathing.
  • If the person becomes responsive, stop CPR and wait for advanced help to arrive.

☐ If the person continues to be unresponsive, continue CPR and use the AED as soon as it is available.

☐ Continue CPR and using the AED until
  • Someone else arrives who can take turns providing CPR with you
  • The person begins to move, speak, blink, or otherwise react
  • Someone with more advanced training arrives

CPR and AED Use for Children

What You Will Learn   In this section, you will learn when CPR is needed, how to give CPR to a child, and how to use an AED.

Definition of a Child   For the purposes of this course, a child is from 1 year of age to puberty. Signs of puberty include chest or underarm hair in males and any breast development in females. If you are in doubt about whether someone is an adult or child, provide emergency care as if the person is an adult.

The definition of *child* is different when using an AED compared with providing CPR. See "Use an AED" later in this section.

Pediatric Chain of Survival   The AHA pediatric Chain of Survival (Figure 42) shows the most important actions needed to treat cardiac arrests in children that occur outside of a hospital.

During this course, you will learn about the first 3 links of the chain. The fourth and fifth links are advanced care provided by emergency responders and hospital providers who will take over care.

First link 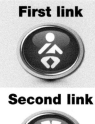	Preventing injury and sudden cardiac arrest is an important first step in saving children's lives.
Second link	The sooner that high-quality CPR is started for someone in cardiac arrest, the better the chances of survival.
Third link	Phoning 9-1-1 as soon as possible so that the child can have emergency care quickly improves outcome.

Remember that seconds count when a child has a cardiac arrest. Wherever you are, take action. The pediatric Chain of Survival starts with you!

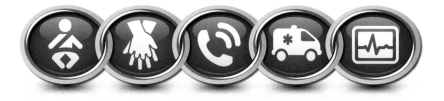

Figure 42. The AHA pediatric Chain of Survival for cardiac arrests outside of a hospital.

Respiratory Problems Often Cause Cardiac Arrest in Children

Children usually have healthy hearts. Breathing trouble is often the cause of a child needing CPR. In the pediatric Chain of Survival, preventing cardiac arrest is one of the most important things you can do. This includes prevention of drowning, choking, and other respiratory problems.

Because respiratory problems are often the cause of cardiac arrest in children, if you are alone and do not have a phone nearby, provide CPR for 2 minutes before leaving to phone 9-1-1.

Topics Covered

- Assess and phone 9-1-1
- Perform high-quality CPR
- Use an AED
- Putting it all together: child high-quality CPR AED summary

When you encounter a child who may have had a cardiac arrest, take the following steps to assess the emergency and get help:

- Make sure the scene is safe.
- Tap and shout (check for responsiveness).
- Shout for help.
- Check for breathing.
- Phone 9-1-1, begin CPR, and get an AED.

Depending on the particular circumstance and the resources you have available, you may be able to perform some of these actions at the same time. You might, for example, phone 9-1-1 with your cell phone on speaker mode while checking for breathing.

Make Sure the Scene Is Safe

Before you assess the child, make sure the scene is safe. Look for anything nearby that might hurt you. You can't help if you get hurt too.

As you give care, be aware if anything changes and makes it unsafe for you or the child.

Tap and Shout (Check for Responsiveness)

Tap and shout to check if the child is responsive or unresponsive (Figure 43). Lean over the child or kneel at his side. Tap his shoulders and ask if he is OK.

If	Then
The child moves, speaks, blinks, or otherwise reacts when you tap him.	• He is *responsive*. • Ask the child if he needs help.
The child doesn't move, speak, blink, or otherwise react when you tap him.	• He is *unresponsive*. • Shout for help so that if others are nearby, they can help you.

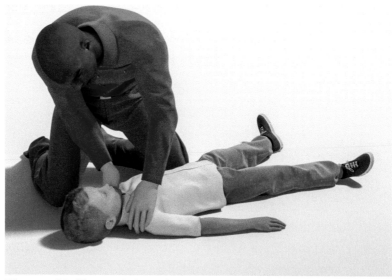

Figure 43. Tap and shout (check for responsiveness).

Shout for Help

In an emergency, the sooner you realize that there's a problem and get additional help, the better it is for the child with a cardiac arrest.

If the child is unresponsive, shout for help (Figure 44). If someone comes, send that person to phone 9-1-1 and get an AED. If you have a cell phone, phone 9-1-1 and put it on speaker mode.

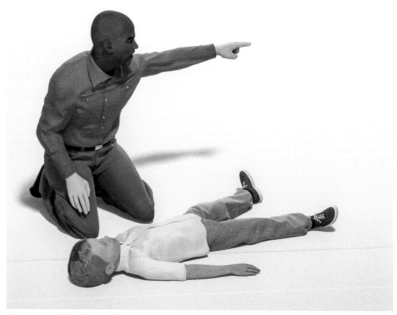

Figure 44. Shout for help.

Check for Breathing   If the child is unresponsive, check for breathing (Figure 45).

Scan the child from head to chest repeatedly for at least 5 seconds (but no more than 10 seconds) looking for chest rise and fall. If the child is not breathing or is only gasping, he needs CPR. (See "Heartsaver Pediatric First Aid CPR AED Terms and Concepts" for more information on gasping.)

If	Then
The child is unresponsive and is breathing.	• This child does not need CPR. • Roll him onto his side (if you don't think he has a neck or back injury). This will help keep the airway clear in the event the child vomits. • If no one has done so, phone 9-1-1, and then return to the child. • If the child is having breathing problems, help him. See "Breathing Problems (Asthma)" in Part 2. • Stay with the child until advanced help arrives.
The child is unresponsive and not breathing or is only gasping.	• This child needs CPR. • If you are alone with no cell phone, give 5 sets of 30 compressions and 2 breaths. • Then, if no one has done so, phone 9-1-1 and get an AED. Return to the child. • Resume CPR and using the AED until advanced help arrives and takes over.

Remember

Unresponsive
+
No breathing
or only gasping

=

Provide CPR

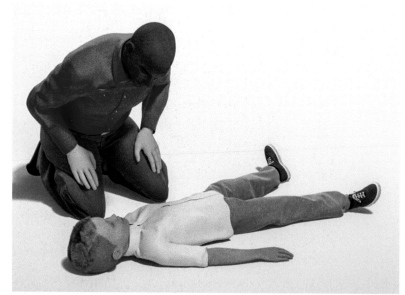

Figure 45. Check for breathing.

Phone 9-1-1, Begin CPR, and Get an AED

If someone comes in response to your shout for help and a cell phone is available

- Ask the person to phone 9-1-1 and get an AED. Ask that the phone be placed on speaker mode so that you can hear the dispatcher's instructions.
- Check the child's breathing, and begin CPR if needed.

If someone comes in response to your shout for help and a cell phone is not available

- Send the person to go phone 9-1-1 and get an AED.
- Check the child's breathing, and begin CPR if needed.

If you are alone and have a cell phone or nearby phone

- Phone 9-1-1. Put the phone on speaker mode so that you can hear the dispatcher's instructions while you continue providing emergency care.
- Check the child's breathing, and begin CPR if needed.
  - Give 5 sets of 30 compressions and 2 breaths.
  - Go get an AED, and return to the child.
  - Resume CPR and using the AED until advanced help arrives and takes over.

If you are alone and don't have a cell phone

- Check the child's breathing, and begin CPR if needed.
  - Give 5 sets of 30 compressions and 2 breaths.
  - Go phone 9-1-1, and get an AED. Return to the child.
  - Resume CPR and using the AED until advanced help arrives and takes over.

Follow Dispatcher's Instructions

Stay on the phone until the 9-1-1 dispatcher tells you to hang up. Answering the dispatcher's questions will not delay the arrival of help.

The dispatcher will ask you about the emergency—where you are and what has happened. Dispatchers can provide instructions that will help you, such as telling you how to provide CPR, use an AED, or give first aid.

That's why it's important to put the phone on speaker mode after phoning 9-1-1 so that the dispatcher and the person providing CPR can speak to each other.

What to Do If You Are Not Sure

If you think a child needs CPR but you aren't sure, provide CPR because you may save a life. CPR is not likely to cause harm if the child is not in cardiac arrest.

It's better to give CPR to a child who doesn't need it than not to give it to a child who does need it.

Summary

Here is a summary of how to assess the emergency and get help when you encounter an ill or injured child:

Assess and Get Help

☐ Make sure the scene is safe.

☐ Tap and shout (check for responsiveness).
  • If the child is *responsive*, you need to find the problem. See "Find the Problem" in Part 1.
  • If the child is *unresponsive*, go to the next steps.

☐ Shout for help.
  • If someone comes, send that person to phone 9-1-1 and get an AED.
  • If you have a cell phone, phone 9-1-1 and put it on speaker mode.

☐ Check for breathing.
  • If the child is unresponsive but breathing, he doesn't need CPR.
    – Roll him onto his side (if you don't think he has a neck or back injury).
    – If no one has done so, phone 9-1-1.
    – Stay with the child until advanced help arrives.
  • If the child is unresponsive and *not* breathing or is only gasping, begin CPR and use an AED. See the next steps.

☐ *If someone comes in response to your shout for help and a cell phone is available*

- Ask the person to phone 9-1-1 and get an AED. Ask that the phone be placed on speaker mode so that you can hear the dispatcher's instructions.
- Check the child's breathing, and begin CPR if needed.

☐ *If someone comes in response to your shout for help and a cell phone is not available*

- Send the person to go phone 9-1-1 and get an AED.
- Check the child's breathing, and begin CPR if needed.

☐ *If you are alone and have a cell phone or nearby phone*

- Phone 9-1-1. Put the phone on speaker mode so that you can hear the dispatcher's instructions while you continue providing emergency care.
- Check the child's breathing, and begin CPR if needed.
  - Give 5 sets of 30 compressions and 2 breaths.
  - Go get an AED, and return to the child.
  - Resume CPR and using the AED until advanced help arrives and takes over.

☐ *If you are alone and don't have a cell phone*

- Check the child's breathing, and begin CPR if needed.
  - Give 5 sets of 30 compressions and 2 breaths.
  - Go phone 9-1-1 and get an AED. Return to the child.
  - Resume CPR and using the AED until advanced help arrives and takes over.

☐ Continue providing CPR and using the AED until
- Someone else arrives who can take turns providing CPR with you
- The child begins to move, speak, blink, or otherwise react
- Someone with more advanced training arrives

Perform High-Quality CPR

Learning how to perform high-quality CPR is important. The better the CPR skills are performed, the better the chances of survival.

CPR Skills

CPR has 2 main skills:

- Providing compressions
- Giving breaths

You will learn how to perform these skills for a child in cardiac arrest in this section.

Provide Compressions

A compression is the act of pushing hard and fast on the chest. When a child's heart stops, blood stops flowing through the body. When you push on the chest, you pump blood to the brain and heart.

To perform high-quality compressions, make sure that you

- Provide compressions that are deep enough
- Provide compressions that are fast enough
- Let the chest come back up to its normal position after each compression
- Try not to interrupt compressions for more than 10 seconds, even when you give breaths

Compression depth is an important part of providing high-quality compressions. You need to push hard enough to pump blood through the body. It's better to push too hard than not hard enough. People are often afraid of causing a child injury by providing compressions, but injury is unlikely.

Compression Technique

When providing compressions for a child, use 1 hand (Figure 46). If you can't push down at least one third the depth of the child's chest (or about 2 inches) with 1 hand, use 2 hands to compress the chest (Figure 47).

Here is how to provide compressions for a child during CPR:

How to Provide Compressions for a Child During CPR
☐ Make sure the child is lying on his back on a firm, flat surface.
☐ Quickly move clothes out of the way.
☐ Use either 1 hand or 2 hands to give compressions.
• **1 hand:** Put the heel of one hand on the center of the chest (over the lower half of the breastbone).   • **2 hands:** Put the heel of one hand on the center of the chest (over the lower half of the breastbone). Put your other hand on top of the first hand.
☐ Push straight down at least one third the depth of the chest or about 2 inches.
☐ Push at a rate of 100 to 120 compressions per minute. Count the compressions out loud.
☐ Let the chest come back up to its normal position after each compression.

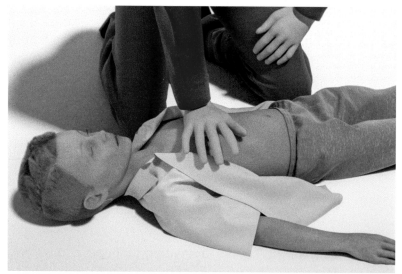

Figure 46. Using 1 hand to give compressions to a child.

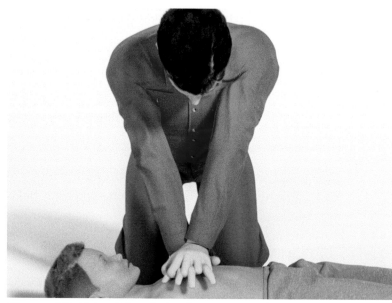

Figure 47. Using 2 hands to give compressions to a child.

Switch Rescuers to Avoid Fatigue

Performing chest compressions correctly is hard work. The more tired you become, the less effective your compressions will be.

If someone else knows CPR, you can take turns providing CPR (Figure 48). Switch rescuers about every 2 minutes, or sooner if you get tired, moving quickly to keep any pauses in compressions as short as possible.

Remind other rescuers to perform high-quality CPR as described in the table labeled "How to Provide Compressions for a Child During CPR."

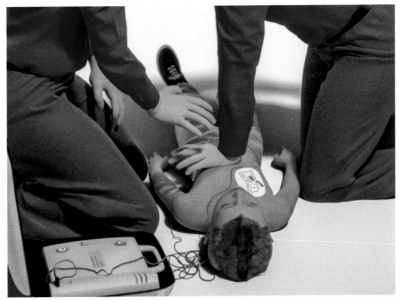

Figure 48. Switch rescuers about every 2 minutes to avoid fatigue.

Give Breaths

The second skill of CPR is giving breaths. After each set of 30 compressions, you will need to give 2 breaths. Breaths may be given with or without a barrier device, such as a pocket mask or face shield.

When you give breaths, the breaths need to make the chest rise visibly. When you can see the chest rise, you know you have delivered an effective breath.

Open the Airway

Before giving breaths, open the airway (Figure 49). This lifts the tongue from the back of the throat to make sure your breaths get air into the lungs.

Follow these steps to open the airway:

How to Open the Airway
☐ Put one hand on the forehead and the fingers of your other hand on the bony part of the chin (Figure 49).
☐ Tilt the head back and lift the chin.

Avoid pressing into the soft part of the neck or under the chin because this might block the airway.

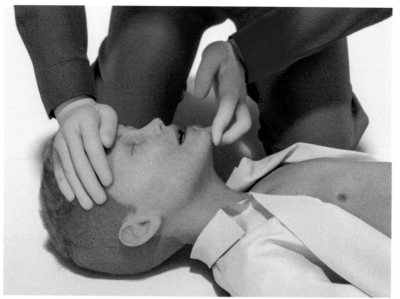

Figure 49. Open the airway by tilting the head back and lifting the chin.

Give Breaths Without a Pocket Mask

If you choose to give someone breaths without a barrier device, it is usually quite safe because there is very little chance that you will catch a disease.

As you give each breath, look at the child's chest to see if it begins to rise. For small children, you will not need to blow as much as for larger children. Actually seeing the chest begin to rise is the best way to know that your breaths are effective.

Follow these steps to give breaths without a pocket mask or face shield (Figure 50):

How to Give Breaths Without a Mask
☐ While holding the airway open, pinch the nose closed with your thumb and forefinger.
☐ Take a normal breath. Cover the child's mouth with your mouth.
☐ Give 2 breaths (blow for 1 second for each). Watch for the chest to begin to rise as you give each breath.
☐ Try not to interrupt compressions for more than 10 seconds.

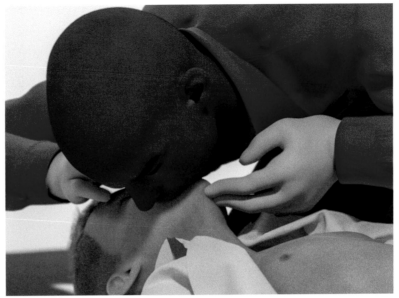

Figure 50. Cover the child's mouth with your mouth.

What to Do If the Chest Doesn't Rise

It takes a little practice to give breaths correctly. If you give someone a breath and the chest doesn't rise, do the following:

- Allow the head to go back to its normal position.
- Open the airway again by tilting the head back and lifting the chin.
- Then, give another breath. Make sure the chest rises.

Minimize Interruptions in Chest Compressions

If you have been unable to give 2 effective breaths in 10 seconds, go back to pushing hard and fast on the chest. Try to give breaths again after every 30 compressions.

Don't interrupt compressions for more than 10 seconds.

Use a Pocket Mask

You may give breaths with or without a barrier device, such as a pocket mask. Barrier devices are made of plastic and fit over the person's mouth and nose (Figure 51). They protect the rescuer from blood, vomit, or disease. Your instructor may discuss other types of barrier devices, like face shields, which can be used when giving breaths.

If you're in the workplace, your employer may provide personal protective equipment, including pocket masks or face shields, for use during CPR.

There are many different kinds of pocket masks as well as different sizes for adults, children, and infants. So, make sure you're using the right size. You may need to put a pocket mask together before you use it.

Give Breaths With a Pocket Mask

Follow these steps to give breaths with a pocket mask (Figure 51):

<table>
<tr><td>

How to Give Breaths With a Pocket Mask

</td></tr>
<tr><td>

☐ Put the mask over the child's mouth and nose.
- If the mask has a pointed end, put the narrow end of the mask on the bridge of the nose; position the wide end so that it covers the mouth.

</td></tr>
<tr><td>

☐ Tilt the head and lift the chin while pressing the mask against the child's face. It is important to make an airtight seal between the child's face and the mask while you lift the chin to keep the airway open.

</td></tr>
<tr><td>

☐ Give 2 breaths (blow for 1 second for each). Watch for the chest to begin to rise as you give each breath.

</td></tr>
<tr><td>

☐ Try not to interrupt compressions for more than 10 seconds.

</td></tr>
</table>

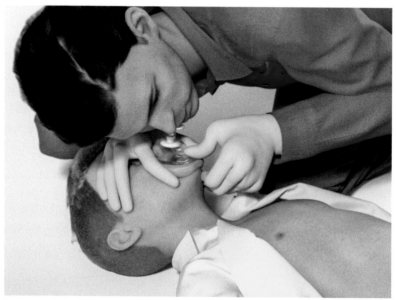

Figure 51. Giving breaths with a pocket mask.

Give Sets of 30 Compressions and 2 Breaths

When providing CPR, give sets of 30 compressions and 2 breaths.

<table>
<tr><td>

How to Give Sets of Compressions and Breaths to a Child

</td></tr>
<tr><td>

☐ Make sure the child is lying on his back on a firm, flat surface.

</td></tr>
<tr><td>

☐ Quickly move clothes out of the way.

</td></tr>
</table>

(continued)

(continued)

☐ Give 30 chest compressions.
- Use either 1 hand or 2 hands to give compressions.
- **1 hand:** Put the heel of one hand on the center of the chest (over the lower half of the breastbone).
- **2 hands:** Put the heel of one hand on the center of the chest (over the lower half of the breastbone). Put your other hand on top of the first hand.
- Push straight down at least one third the depth of the chest or about 2 inches.
- Push at a rate of 100 to 120 compressions per minute. Count the compressions out loud.
- Let the chest come back up to its normal position after each compression.

☐ After 30 compressions, give 2 breaths.
- Open the airway and give 2 breaths (blow for 1 second for each). Watch for the chest to begin to rise as you give each breath.
- Try not to interrupt compressions for more than 10 seconds.

Use an AED

CPR combined with using an AED provides the best chance of saving a life. If possible, use an AED every time you provide CPR.

AEDs can be used for children and infants, as well as adults.

- Some AEDs can deliver a smaller shock dose for children and infants if you use child pads or a child-cable key or switch.
- If the AED can deliver the smaller shock dose, use it for infants and children less than 8 years of age.
- If the AED cannot deliver a child shock dose, you can use the adult pads and give an adult shock dose for infants and children less than 8 years of age.

AEDs are safe, accurate, and easy to use. Once you turn on the AED, follow the prompts. The AED will analyze if the child needs a shock and will automatically give one or tell you when to give one.

Turn on the AED

To use an AED, turn it on by either pushing the "on" button or lifting the lid (Figure 52). Once you turn on the AED, you will hear prompts, which will tell you everything you need to do.

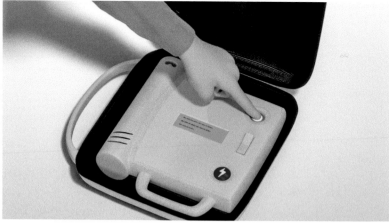

Figure 52. Turning on the AED.

Attach the Pads

Many AEDs have pads for adults and a child pad-cable system or key for children and infants.

- Use child pads if the child or infant is less than 8 years old. If child pads are not available, use adult pads.
- Use adult pads if the child is 8 years old or older.

Before you place the pads, quickly scan the child to see if there are any special situations that might require additional steps. See "Special Situations" later in this section.

Peel away the backing from the pads. Follow the pad placement as shown on the images on the pads or package. Attach the pads to the child's bare chest (Figure 53).

When you put the pads on the chest, make sure they don't touch each other. If the child's chest is small, the pads may overlap. In this case you may need to put one pad on the child's chest and the other on the child's back.

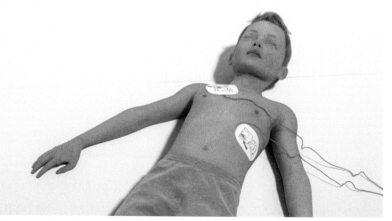

Figure 53. Place pads on a child by following the pictures on the pads.

Clear the Child If a Shock Is Advised

Let the AED analyze the heart rhythm. If the AED advises a shock, it will tell you to stay clear of the child. If so, then loudly state, "Clear." Make sure that no one is touching the child just before you push the "shock" button (Figure 54).

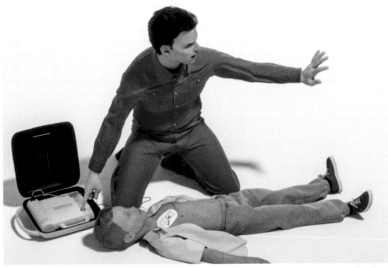

Figure 54. Make sure that no one is touching the child just before you push the "shock" button.

Steps for Using the AED for a Child

Use the AED as soon as it is available. Here are the steps for using the AED for a child:

How to Use an AED for a Child

☐ Turn the AED on and follow the prompts.
- Turn it on by pushing the "on" button or lifting the lid (Figure 52).
- Follow the prompts, which will tell you everything you need to do.

☐ Attach the pads.
- Use child pads if the child is less than 8 years old. If child pads are not available, use adult pads.
- Use adult pads if the child is 8 years old or older.
- Peel away the backing from the pads.
- Following the pictures on the pads, attach them to the child's bare chest (Figure 53). Make sure the pads don't touch each other.

☐ Let the AED analyze.
- Loudly state, "Clear," and make sure that no one is touching the child.
- The AED will analyze the heart rhythm.
- If a shock is not needed, resume CPR.

☐ Deliver a shock if needed (Figure 54).
- Loudly state, "Clear," and make sure that no one is touching the child.
- Push the "shock" button.
- Immediately resume CPR.

Special Situations

There are some special situations that you may need to consider before placing AED pads. Although it is not very common, you may encounter a medicine patch or a device on a child, which may interfere with the AED pad placement.

Quickly scan the child to see if he has any of the following *before* applying the pads:

If the child...	Then
Is lying in water	• Quickly move the child to a dry area.
Is lying on snow or in a small puddle	• You may use the AED (the chest doesn't have to be completely dry). • If the chest is covered with water or sweat, quickly wipe it before attaching the pads.
Has water on the chest	• Quickly wipe the chest dry before attaching the pads.
Has an implanted defibrillator or pacemaker	• Don't put the AED pad directly over the implanted device. • Follow the normal steps for operating an AED.
Has a medicine patch where you need to place an AED pad	• Don't put the AED pad directly over a medicine patch. • Use protective gloves. • Remove the medicated patch. • Wipe the area clean. • Attach the AED pads.

Continue Providing CPR and Using the AED

As soon as the AED gives the shock, immediately resume chest compressions. Continue to follow the AED prompts, which will guide the rescue.

Provide CPR and use the AED until

- Someone else arrives who can take turns providing CPR with you
- The child begins to move, speak, blink, or otherwise react
- Someone with more advanced training arrives

Putting It All Together: Child High-Quality CPR AED Summary

Children usually have healthy hearts. Often, a child's heart stops because the child can't breathe or is having trouble breathing. As a result, it's very important to give breaths as well as compressions to a child.

Compressions are still very important to deliver blood flow and are the core of CPR. Try not to interrupt chest compressions for more than 10 seconds when you give breaths.

☐ Make sure the scene is safe.

☐ Tap and shout (check for responsiveness).
- If the child is *responsive*, you need to find the problem. See "Find the Problem" in Part 1.
- If the child is *unresponsive*, go to the next steps.

☐ Shout for help.
- If someone comes, send that person to phone 9-1-1 and get an AED.
- If you have a cell phone, phone 9-1-1 and put it on speaker mode.

☐ Check for breathing.
- If the child is unresponsive but breathing, he doesn't need CPR.
  - Roll him onto his side (if you don't think he has a neck or back injury).
  - If no one has done so, phone 9-1-1.
  - Stay with the child until advanced help arrives.
- If the child is unresponsive and *not* breathing or only gasping, begin CPR and use the AED. See the next steps.

Phone 9-1-1, Begin CPR, and Get an AED

☐ *If someone comes in response to your shout for help and a cell phone is available*
- Ask the person to phone 9-1-1 and get an AED. Ask that the phone be placed on speaker mode so that you can hear the dispatcher's instructions.
- Check the child's breathing, and begin CPR if needed.

☐ *If someone comes in response to your shout for help and a cell phone is not available*
- Send the person to go phone 9-1-1 and get an AED.
- Check the child's breathing, and begin CPR if needed.

☐ *If you are alone and have a cell phone or nearby phone*
- Phone 9-1-1. Put the phone on speaker mode so that you can hear the dispatcher's instructions while you continue providing emergency care.
- Check the child's breathing, and begin CPR if needed.
  - Give 5 sets of 30 compressions and 2 breaths.
  - Go get an AED, and return to the child.
  - Resume CPR and using the AED until advanced help arrives and takes over.

(continued)

(continued)

Phone 9-1-1, Begin CPR, and Get an AED

☐ *If you are alone and don't have a cell phone*
  - Check the child's breathing, and begin CPR if needed.
    - Give 5 sets of 30 compressions and 2 breaths.
    - Go phone 9-1-1, and get an AED. Return to the child.
    - Resume CPR and using the AED until advanced help arrives and takes over.

Provide High-Quality CPR

When providing CPR, you give sets of 30 compressions and 2 breaths.

☐ Make sure the child is lying on his back on a firm, flat surface.

☐ Quickly move clothes out of the way.

☐ Give 30 chest compressions.
  - Use either 1 hand or 2 hands to give compressions.
    - **1 hand:** Put the heel of one hand on the center of the chest (over the lower half of the breastbone).
    - **2 hands:** Put the heel of one hand on the center of the chest (over the lower half of the breastbone). Put your other hand on top of the first hand.
  - Push straight down at least one third the depth of the chest or about 2 inches.
  - Push at a rate of 100 to 120 compressions per minute. Count the compressions out loud.
  - Let the chest come back up to its normal position after each compression.

☐ After 30 compressions, give 2 breaths.
  - Open the airway and give 2 breaths (blow for 1 second for each). Watch for the chest to begin to rise as you give each breath.
  - Try not to interrupt compressions for more than 10 seconds.

☐ Use an AED as soon as it is available.
  - Turn the AED on and follow the prompts.
  - Attach the pads.
    - Use child pads if the child is less than 8 years old. If child pads are not available, use adult pads.
    - Use adult pads if the child is 8 years old or older.
  - Let the AED analyze.
  - Make sure no one is touching the child, and deliver a shock if advised.

(continued)

Provide High-Quality CPR

☐ Provide CPR and use the AED until
- Someone else arrives who can take turns providing CPR with you
- The child begins to move, speak, blink, or otherwise react
- Someone with more advanced training arrives and takes over

CPR for Infants

What You Will Learn

In this section, you will learn when CPR is needed, how to give CPR to an infant, and how to use an AED.

Definition of an Infant

For the purposes of this course, an infant is less than 1 year old.

Differences in CPR Between an Infant and a Child

Because infants are so small, there are some differences between infants, children, and adults in how CPR is performed. When providing compressions on an infant, you use only 2 fingers of 1 hand—vs 1 or 2 hands for a child and 2 hands for an adult.

Also, for an infant, you should push down about 1½ inches at the rate of 100 to 120 compressions per minute.

Topics Covered

- Assess and phone 9-1-1
- Perform high-quality CPR
- Use an AED
- Putting it all together: infant high-quality CPR summary

Assess and Phone 9-1-1

When you encounter an infant who may have had a cardiac arrest, take the following steps to assess the emergency and get help:

- Make sure the scene is safe.
- Tap and shout (check for responsiveness).
- Shout for help.
- Check for breathing.
- Phone 9-1-1, begin CPR, and get an AED.

Depending on the particular circumstance and the resources you have available, you may be able to perform some of these actions at the same time. You might, for example, phone 9-1-1 with your cell phone on speaker mode while checking for breathing.

Make Sure the Scene Is Safe

Before you assess the infant, make sure the scene is safe. Look for anything nearby that might hurt you. You can't help if you get hurt too.

As you give care, be aware if anything changes and makes it unsafe for you or the infant.

Tap and Shout (Check for Responsiveness)

Tap and shout to check if the infant is responsive or unresponsive (Figure 55). Tap the infant's foot and shout his name.

If	Then
The infant moves, cries, blinks, or otherwise reacts when you tap him.	• He is *responsive*; continue first aid care.
The infant doesn't move, cry, blink, or otherwise react when you tap him.	• He is *unresponsive*. • Shout for help so that if others are nearby, they can help you.

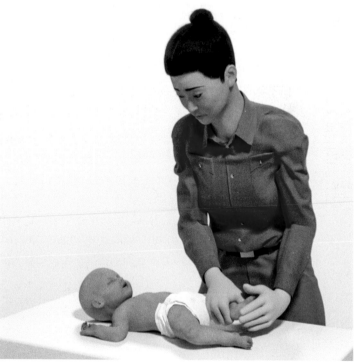

Figure 55. Tap and shout (check for responsiveness).

Shout for Help

In an emergency, the sooner you realize that there's a problem and get additional help, the better it is for the infant with a cardiac arrest. When more people are helping, you are able to provide better care to the infant.

If the infant is unresponsive, shout for help (Figure 56). If someone comes, send that person to phone 9-1-1 and get an AED. If you have a cell phone, phone 9-1-1 and put it on speaker mode.

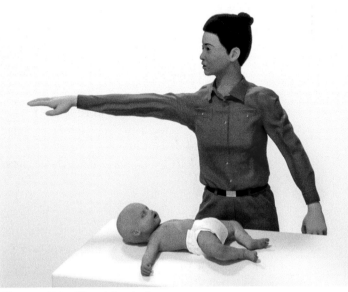

Figure 56. Shout for help.

Check for Breathing

If the infant is unresponsive, check for breathing (Figure 57).

Scan the infant from head to chest repeatedly for at least 5 seconds (but no more than 10 seconds) looking for chest rise and fall. If the infant is not breathing or is only gasping, he needs CPR. (See "Heartsaver Pediatric First Aid CPR AED Terms and Concepts" for more information on gasping.)

If	Then
The infant is unresponsive and is breathing.	• This infant does not need CPR. • Roll him onto his side (if you don't think he has a neck or back injury). This will help keep the airway clear in the event the infant vomits. • If no one has done so, phone 9-1-1, and then return to the infant. • If the infant is having breathing problems, help him. See "Breathing Problems (Asthma)" in Part 2. • Stay with the infant until advanced help arrives.
The infant is unresponsive and not breathing or is only gasping.	• This infant needs CPR. • If you are alone with no cell phone, give 5 sets of 30 compressions and 2 breaths. • Then, if no one has done so, phone 9-1-1 and get an AED. Return to the infant. • Resume CPR and using the AED until advanced help arrives and takes over.

Remember

Unresponsive
+
No breathing
or only gasping

=

**Provide
CPR**

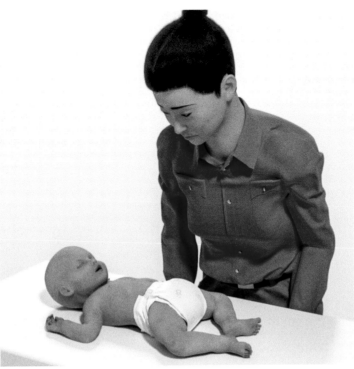

Figure 57. Check for breathing.

Phone 9-1-1, Begin CPR, and Get an AED

If someone comes in response to your shout for help and a cell phone is available

- Ask the person to phone 9-1-1 and get an AED. Ask that the phone be placed on speaker mode so that you can hear the dispatcher's instructions.
- Check the infant's breathing, and begin CPR if needed.

If someone comes in response to your shout for help and a cell phone is not available

- Send the person to go phone 9-1-1 and get an AED.
- Check the infant's breathing, and begin CPR if needed.

If you are alone and have a cell phone or nearby phone

- Phone 9-1-1. Put the phone on speaker mode so that you can hear the dispatcher's instructions while you continue providing emergency care.
- Give 5 sets of 30 compressions and 2 breaths.
- Go get an AED,* and return to the infant.
- Resume CPR and using the AED until advanced help arrives and takes over.

If you are alone and don't have a cell phone

- Check the infant's breathing, and begin CPR if needed.
- Give 5 sets of 30 compressions and 2 breaths.
- Go phone 9-1-1, and get an AED.* Return to the infant.
- Resume CPR and using the AED until advanced help arrives and takes over.

*If the infant isn't injured and you're alone, after 5 sets of 30 compressions and 2 breaths, you may carry the infant with you to phone 9-1-1 and get an AED (Figure 58).

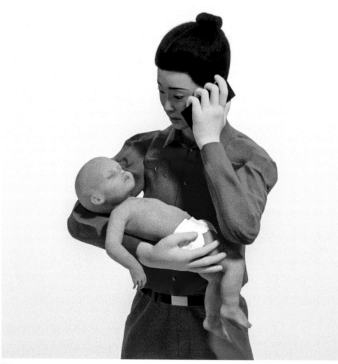

Figure 58. You may carry the infant with you to phone 9-1-1 and get an AED.

Follow Dispatcher's Instructions

Stay on the phone until the 9-1-1 dispatcher tells you to hang up. Answering the dispatcher's questions will not delay the arrival of help.

The dispatcher will ask you about the emergency—where you are and what has happened. Dispatchers can provide instructions that will help you, such as telling you how to provide CPR, use an AED, or give first aid.

That's why it's important to put the phone on speaker mode after phoning 9-1-1 so that the dispatcher and the person providing CPR can speak to each other.

What to Do If You Are Not Sure

If you think an infant needs CPR but you aren't sure, provide CPR because you may save a life. CPR is not likely to cause harm if the infant is not in cardiac arrest.

It's better to give CPR to an infant who doesn't need it than not to give it to an infant who does need it.

Summary

Here is a summary of how to assess the emergency and get help when you encounter an ill or injured infant:

Assess and Get Help

☐ Make sure the scene is safe.

☐ Tap and shout (check for responsiveness).
- If the child is *responsive*, you need to find the problem. See "Find the Problem" in Part 1.
- If the child is *unresponsive*, go to the next steps.

☐ Shout for help.
- If someone comes, send that person to phone 9-1-1 and get an AED.
- If you have a cell phone, phone 9-1-1 and put it on speaker mode.

☐ Check for breathing.
- If the child is unresponsive but breathing, he doesn't need CPR.
  - Roll him onto his side (if you don't think he has a neck or back injury).
  - If no one has done so, phone 9-1-1.
  - Stay with the child until advanced help arrives.
- If the child is unresponsive and *not* breathing or is only gasping, begin CPR and use an AED. See the next steps.

Phone 9-1-1, Begin CPR, and Get an AED

☐ *If someone comes in response to your shout for help and a cell phone is available*
- Ask the person to phone 9-1-1 and get an AED. Ask that the phone be placed on speaker mode so that you can hear the dispatcher's instructions.
- Check the infant's breathing, and begin CPR if needed.

☐ *If someone comes in response to your shout for help and a cell phone is not available*
- Send the person to go phone 9-1-1 and get an AED.
- Check the infant's breathing, and begin CPR if needed.

(continued)

(continued)

☐ *If you are alone and have a cell phone or nearby phone*
- Phone 9-1-1. Put the phone on speaker mode so that you can hear the dispatcher's instructions while you continue providing emergency care.
- Check the infant's breathing, and begin CPR if needed.
- Give 5 sets of 30 compressions and 2 breaths.
- Go get an AED,* and return to the infant.
- Resume CPR and using the AED until advanced help arrives and takes over.

☐ *If you are alone and don't have a cell phone*
- Check the infant's breathing, and begin CPR if needed.
- Give 5 sets of 30 compressions and 2 breaths.
- Go phone 9-1-1, and get an AED.* Return to the infant.
- Resume CPR and using the AED until advanced help arrives and takes over.

*If the infant isn't injured and you're alone, after 5 sets of 30 compressions and 2 breaths, you may carry the infant with you to phone 9-1-1 and get an AED.

☐ Continue providing CPR and using the AED until
- Someone else arrives who can take turns providing CPR with you
- The infant begins to move, speak, blink, or otherwise react
- Someone with more advanced training arrives

Perform High-Quality CPR

Learning how to perform high-quality CPR is important. The better the CPR skills are performed, the better the chances of survival.

CPR Skills

CPR has 2 main skills:

- Providing compressions
- Giving breaths

You will learn how to perform these skills for an infant in cardiac arrest in this section.

Provide Compressions

A compression is the act of pushing hard and fast on the chest. When an infant's heart stops, blood stops flowing through the body. When you push on the chest, you pump blood to the brain and heart.

Pushing hard and fast when providing compressions is just as important with infants as it is with children and adults.

Compressions are the most important part of CPR. To perform high-quality CPR, make sure that you

- Provide compressions that are deep enough
- Provide compressions that are fast enough
- Let the chest come back up to its normal position after each compression
- Try not to interrupt compressions for more than 10 seconds, even when you give breaths

Compression depth is an important part of providing high-quality compressions. You need to push hard enough to pump blood through the body. It's better to push too hard than not hard enough. People are often afraid of causing an infant injury by providing compressions, but injury is unlikely.

Compression Technique

One of the main differences in infant CPR is that you use just 2 fingers in providing compressions. Look at Figure 59 to see the correct placement of your fingers on the baby's chest. Place 2 fingers of 1 hand on the breastbone, just below the nipple line. Push straight down at least one third the depth of the chest or about 1½ inches.

Here is how to provide compressions for an infant during CPR:

How to Provide Compressions for an Infant During CPR
☐ Make sure the infant is lying on his back on a firm, flat surface.
☐ Quickly move clothes out of the way.
☐ Use 2 fingers of 1 hand to give compressions. Place them on the breastbone, just below the nipple line (Figure 59).
☐ Push straight down at least one third the depth of the chest or about 1½ inches.
☐ Push at a rate of 100 to 120 compressions per minute. Count the compressions out loud.
☐ Let the chest come back up to its normal position after each compression.

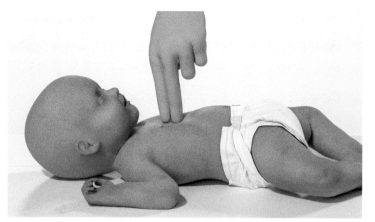

Figure 59. Use 2 fingers of 1 hand to give compressions. Place them on the breastbone, just below the nipple line. Avoid the tip of the breastbone.

Switch Rescuers to Avoid Fatigue

Performing chest compressions correctly is hard work. The more tired you become, the less effective your compressions will be.

If someone else knows CPR, you can take turns providing CPR. Switch rescuers about every 2 minutes, or sooner if you get tired, moving quickly to keep any pauses in compressions as short as possible.

Remind other rescuers to perform high-quality CPR as described in the table labeled "How to Provide Compressions for an Infant During CPR."

Give Breaths

The second skill of CPR is giving breaths. After each set of 30 compressions, you will need to give 2 breaths. Breaths may be given with or without a barrier device, such as a pocket mask or face shield.

Infants often have healthy hearts, but even an infant's heart can stop beating if he can't breathe or has trouble breathing. So, it's very important to give breaths as well as compressions to an infant who needs CPR.

When you give breaths, the breaths need to make the chest rise visibly. When you can see the chest rise, you know you have delivered an effective breath.

Before giving breaths, open the airway. This lifts the tongue from the back of the throat to make sure your breaths get air into the lungs.

Opening the infant's airway too far can actually *close* the infant's airway, making it difficult to get air inside. Follow these steps to make sure you open the infant's airway correctly:

How to Open the Airway

☐ Put one hand on the forehead and the fingers of your other hand on the bony part of the chin.

☐ Tilt the head back and lift the chin.

Avoid pressing into the soft part of the neck or under the chin because this might block the airway. Also, don't push the head back too far. This might close the airway as well.

Give Breaths Without a Pocket Mask

If you choose to give someone breaths without a barrier device, it is usually quite safe because there is very little chance that you will catch a disease.

As you give each breath, look at the infant's chest to see if it begins to rise. You will not need to blow as much as for a larger child. Actually seeing the chest begin to rise is the best way to know that your breaths are effective.

Follow these steps to give breaths without a pocket mask or face shield (Figure 60):

How to Give Breaths Without a Pocket Mask

☐ While holding the airway open, take a normal breath. Cover the infant's mouth and nose with your mouth. If you have difficulty making an effective seal, try either a mouth-to-mouth or a mouth-to-nose breath.
  • If you use the mouth-to-mouth technique, pinch the nose closed.
  • If you use the mouth-to-nose technique, close the mouth.

☐ Give 2 breaths (blow for 1 second for each). Watch for the chest to begin to rise as you give each breath.

☐ Try not to interrupt compressions for more than 10 seconds.

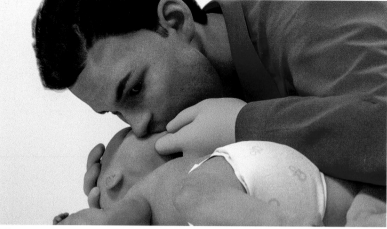

Figure 60. Cover the infant's mouth and nose with your mouth.

What to Do If the Chest Doesn't Rise

It takes a little practice to give breaths correctly. If you give someone a breath and the chest doesn't rise, do the following:

- Allow the head to go back to its normal position.
- Open the airway again by tilting the head back and lifting the chin.
- Then, give another breath. Make sure the chest rises.

Minimize Interruptions in Chest Compressions

If you have been unable to give 2 effective breaths in 10 seconds, go back to pushing hard and fast on the chest. Try to give breaths again after every 30 compressions.

Don't interrupt compressions for more than 10 seconds.

Use a Pocket Mask

You may give breaths with or without a barrier device, such as a pocket mask. Barrier devices are made of plastic and fit over the person's mouth and nose (Figure 61). They protect the rescuer from blood, vomit, or disease. Your instructor may discuss other types of barrier devices, like face shields, which can be used when giving breaths.

If you're in the workplace, your employer may provide personal protective equipment, including pocket masks or face shields, for use during CPR.

There are many different kinds of pocket masks as well as different sizes for adults, children, and infants. So, make sure you're using the right size. You may need to put a pocket mask together before you use it.

Give Breaths With a Pocket Mask

Follow these steps to give breaths with a pocket mask (Figure 61):

How to Give Breaths With a Pocket Mask

☐ Put the mask over the infant's mouth and nose.
  • If the mask has a pointed end, put the narrow end of the mask on the bridge of the nose; position the wide end so that it covers the mouth.

☐ Tilt the head and lift the chin while pressing the mask against the infant's face. It is important to make an airtight seal between the infant's face and the mask while you lift the chin to keep the airway open.

☐ Give 2 breaths (blow for 1 second for each). Watch for the chest to begin to rise as you give each breath.

☐ Try not to interrupt compressions for more than 10 seconds.

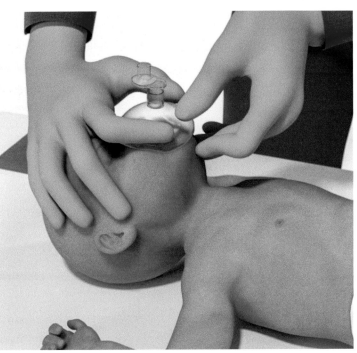

Figure 61. Giving breaths with a pocket mask.

Give Sets of 30 Compressions and 2 Breaths

When providing CPR, give sets of 30 compressions and 2 breaths.

How to Give Sets of Compressions and Breaths to an Infant

☐ Make sure the infant is lying on his back on a firm, flat surface.

☐ Quickly move clothes out of the way.

☐ Give 30 chest compressions.
- Use 2 fingers of 1 hand to give compressions. Place them on the breastbone, just below the nipple line.
- Push straight down at least one third the depth of the chest or about 1½ inches.
- Push at a rate of 100 to 120 compressions per minute. Count the compressions out loud.
- Let the chest come back up to its normal position after each compression.

☐ After 30 compressions, give 2 breaths.
- Open the airway and give 2 breaths (blow for 1 second for each). Watch for the chest to begin to rise as you give each breath.
- Try not to interrupt compressions for more than 10 seconds.

Do Not Delay CPR to Get an AED for an Infant

CPR with both compressions and breaths is the most important thing you can do for an infant in cardiac arrest. Do not delay CPR to get an AED for an infant. If someone brings an AED to you, use it as soon as it arrives. See the "Use an AED" section in "CPR and AED Use for Children."

Putting It All Together: Infant High-Quality CPR Summary

Infants usually have healthy hearts. Often, an infant's heart stops because the infant can't breathe or is having trouble breathing. As a result, it's very important to give breaths as well as compressions to an infant.

Compressions are still very important to deliver blood flow and are the core of CPR. Try not to interrupt chest compressions for more than 10 seconds when you give breaths.

☐ Make sure the scene is safe.

☐ Tap and shout (check for responsiveness).
  - If the child is *responsive*, you need to find the problem. See "Find the Problem" in Part 1.
  - If the child is *unresponsive*, go to the next steps.

☐ Shout for help.
  - If someone comes, send that person to phone 9-1-1 and get an AED.
  - If you have a cell phone, phone 9-1-1 and put it on speaker mode.

☐ Check for breathing.
  - If the child is unresponsive but breathing, he doesn't need CPR.
    - Roll him onto his side (if you don't think he has a neck or back injury).
    - If no one has done so, phone 9-1-1.
    - Stay with the child until advanced help arrives.
  - If the child is unresponsive and *not* breathing or is only gasping, begin CPR and use an AED. See the next steps.

☐ *If someone comes in response to your shout for help and a cell phone is available*
  - Ask the person to phone 9-1-1 and get an AED. Ask that the phone be placed on speaker mode so that you can hear the dispatcher's instructions.
  - Check the infant's breathing, and begin CPR if needed.

☐ *If someone comes in response to your shout for help and a cell phone is not available*
  - Send the person to go phone 9-1-1 and get an AED.
  - Check the infant's breathing, and begin CPR if needed.

☐ *If you are alone and have a cell phone or nearby phone*
  - Phone 9-1-1. Put the phone on speaker mode so that you can hear the dispatcher's instructions while you continue providing emergency care.
  - Check the infant's breathing, and begin CPR if needed.
  - Give 5 sets of 30 compressions and 2 breaths.
  - Go get an AED,* and return to the infant.
  - Resume CPR and using the AED until advanced help arrives and takes over.

(continued)

(continued)

Phone 9-1-1, Begin CPR, and Get an AED

☐ *If you are alone and don't have a cell phone*
  • Check the infant's breathing, and begin CPR if needed.
  • Give 5 sets of 30 compressions and 2 breaths.
  • Go phone 9-1-1, and get an AED.* Return to the infant.
  • Resume CPR and using the AED until advanced help arrives and takes over.

*If the infant isn't injured and you're alone, after 5 sets of 30 compressions and 2 breaths, you may carry the infant with you to phone 9-1-1 and get an AED.

Provide High-Quality CPR

When providing CPR, you give sets of 30 compressions and 2 breaths.

☐ Make sure the infant is lying on his back on a firm, flat surface.

☐ Quickly move clothes out of the way.

☐ **Give 30 chest compressions.**
  • Use 2 fingers of 1 hand to give compressions. Place them on the breastbone, just below the nipple line.
  • Push straight down at least one third the depth of the chest or about 1½ inches.
  • Push at a rate of 100 to 120 compressions per minute. Count the compressions out loud.
  • Let the chest come back up to its normal position after each compression.

☐ After 30 compressions, give 2 breaths.
  • Open the airway and give 2 breaths (blow for 1 second for each). Watch for the chest to begin to rise as you give each breath.
  • Try not to interrupt compressions for more than 10 seconds.

☐ Use an AED as soon as it is available.
  • Turn the AED on and follow the prompts.
  • Attach the pads.
    – Use child pads for an infant if available.
    – If child pads are not available, use adult pads.
  • Let the AED analyze.
  • Make sure no one is touching the infant, and deliver a shock if advised.

☐ Provide CPR and use the AED until
  • Someone else arrives who can take turns providing CPR with you
  • The infant begins to move, cry, blink, or otherwise react
  • Someone with more advanced training arrives and takes over

How to Help a Choking Adult, Child, or Infant

What You Will Learn In this section, you will learn to assess whether someone has a mild or severe block in the airway and how to take action to help.

Overview Choking is when food or another object gets stuck in the airway in the throat. The object can block the airway and stop air from getting to the lungs.

In adults, choking is often caused by food. In children, choking can be caused by food or an object.

Topics Covered
- Mild vs severe airway block
- How to help an adult, child, or infant with severe airway block
- How to help a choking adult, child, or infant who becomes unresponsive

Mild vs Severe Airway Block

Assess Choking and Take Action The block in the airway that causes choking can be either mild or severe. If the airway block is severe, act quickly. Get the object out so that the person can breathe. Here is how to assess if someone has a mild or severe airway block and what you should do:

	If Someone...	Then Take Action
Mild airway block	• Can talk or make sounds • Can cough loudly	• Stand by and let the person cough. • If you're worried about the person's breathing, phone or send someone to phone 9-1-1.
Severe airway block	• Cannot breathe, talk, or make sounds *or* • Has a cough that has no sound *or* • Makes the choking sign	• Act quickly. • Follow the steps to help an adult, child, or infant with a severe airway block.

The Choking Sign

If someone is choking, he might use the choking sign, which is holding the neck with one or both hands (Figure 62).

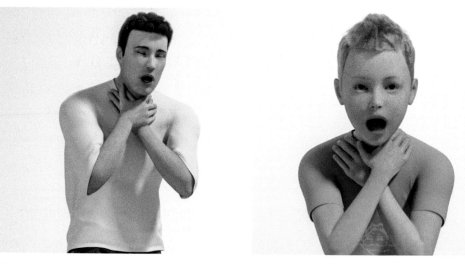

Figure 62. The choking sign: holding the neck with one or both hands.

How to Help an Adult, Child, or Infant With Severe Airway Block

How to Help a Choking Adult or Child With a Severe Airway Block

When an adult or child has a severe airway block, give thrusts slightly above the belly button. These thrusts are called *abdominal thrusts* or the *Heimlich maneuver*. Like a cough, each thrust pushes air from the lungs. This can help move or remove an object that is blocking the airway.

Any person who has received abdominal thrusts should see a healthcare provider as soon as possible.

Follow these steps to help a choking adult or child with a severe airway block.

How to Help a Choking Adult or Child With a Severe Airway Block

☐ If you think someone is choking, ask, "Are you choking? Can I help you?"

☐ If the person nods yes, tell him you are going to help.

☐ Stand firmly or kneel behind the person (depending on your size and the size of the person choking). Wrap your arms around the person's waist so that your fists are in front.

☐ Make a fist with one hand.

☐ Put the thumb side of your fist slightly above the person's belly button and well below the breastbone.

☐ Grasp the fist with your other hand and give quick upward thrusts into the abdomen (Figure 63).

☐ Give thrusts until the object is forced out and the person can breathe, cough, or speak, or until he becomes unresponsive.

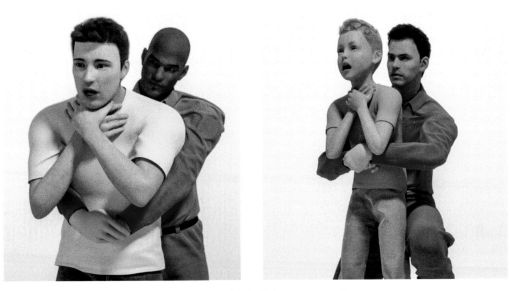

Figure 63. Giving abdominal thrusts (Heimlich maneuver).

How to Help a Choking Pregnant Woman or Large Adult or Child With a Severe Airway Block

If the person with severe airway block is pregnant or very large, give chest thrusts instead of abdominal thrusts.

Follow these steps to help a pregnant woman or large person with a severe airway block:

How to Help a Choking Pregnant Woman or Large Adult or Child With a Severe Airway Block
☐ If you can't wrap your arms fully around the waist, give thrusts on the chest (chest thrusts) instead of on the abdomen.
☐ Put your arms under the person's armpits and your hands on the lower half of the breastbone.
☐ Pull straight back to give chest thrusts (Figure 64).

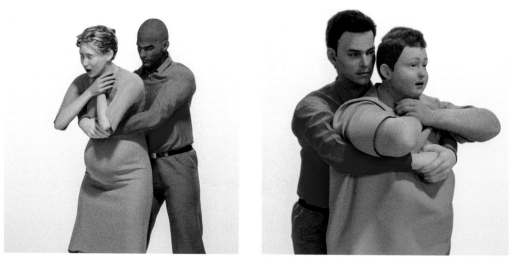

Figure 64. Giving chest thrusts to a pregnant woman or large adult or child with severe airway block.

How to Help a Choking Infant With Severe Airway Block

When an infant has a severe airway block, use back slaps and chest thrusts to help remove the object. *Give only back slaps and chest thrusts to an infant who is choking.* Giving thrusts to an infant's abdomen can cause serious harm.

Follow these steps to help an infant with a severe airway block:

How to Help a Choking Infant With a Severe Airway Block
☐ Hold the infant facedown on your forearm. Support the infant's head and jaw with your hand.
☐ Give up to 5 back slaps with the heel of your other hand, between the infant's shoulder blades (Figure 65A).

(continued)

(continued)

How to Help a Choking Infant With a Severe Airway Block

☐ If the object does not come out after 5 back slaps, turn the infant onto his back, supporting the head.

☐ Give up to 5 chest thrusts, using 2 fingers of your other hand to push on the chest in the same place you push during CPR (Figure 65B).

☐ Repeat giving 5 back slaps and 5 chest thrusts until the infant can breathe, cough, or cry, or until he becomes unresponsive.

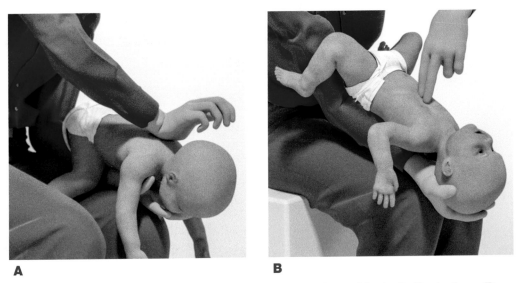

A **B**

Figure 65. How to help an infant who has a severe airway block. **A**, Back slaps. **B**, Chest thrusts.

How to Help a Choking Adult, Child, or Infant Who Becomes Unresponsive

If you can't remove the object blocking the airway, the person will become unresponsive. Always give CPR to anyone who is unresponsive and not breathing normally or only gasping. Giving both compressions and breaths is very important for someone with severe airway block who becomes unresponsive.

Remember	Unresponsive + No breathing or only gasping	=	Provide CPR + Remove object in mouth, if possible

How to Help a Choking Adult Who Becomes Unresponsive

Follow these steps to help an adult with a severe airway block who becomes unresponsive:

How to Help a Choking Adult Who Becomes Unresponsive

☐ Shout for help.

☐ Phone or have someone phone 9-1-1 and get an AED. Put the phone on speaker mode so that you can talk to the dispatcher.

☐ Provide CPR, starting with compressions.

☐ After each set of 30 compressions, open the airway to give breaths.

☐ Look in the mouth. If you see an object in the mouth, take it out.

☐ Give 2 breaths and then repeat 30 compressions.

☐ Continue CPR until
  • The person moves, speaks, blinks, or otherwise reacts
  • Someone with more advanced training arrives and takes over

Remember

Every time you open the airway to give breaths, look for the object in the back of the throat. If you see an object in the mouth, take it out.

Do not perform a blind finger sweep. This could cause the object to get lodged further back in the airway.

How to Help a Child or Infant With a Severe Airway Block Who Becomes Unresponsive

A child or infant who has a severe airway block and becomes unresponsive needs immediate CPR. If you are alone without a cell phone, it is important to provide 5 sets of 30 compressions and 2 breaths first. Each time you give breaths, you need to look in the mouth and remove any object that you see. After the 5 sets of compressions and breaths, if you have no cell phone, leave the child, or take the infant with you, to phone 9-1-1 and get an AED if one is available.

Continue giving sets of 30 compressions and 2 breaths, looking in the mouth after each set of 30 compressions until you can remove the object. Then continue compressions and breaths until the AED arrives, the child or infant responds, or someone with more advanced training arrives and takes over.

Follow these steps to help a choking child or infant with a severe airway block who becomes unresponsive:

How to Help a Choking Child or Infant Who Becomes Unresponsive

☐ Shout for help. Make sure the child or infant is lying on his back on a firm, flat surface.

☐ Begin CPR, phone 9-1-1, and get an AED.

If a cell phone is available

- Phone 9-1-1 on the cell phone; put it on speaker mode while you begin CPR.

If someone comes to help

- Send the person to phone 9-1-1 and get an AED while you begin CPR.

If you are alone and without a phone

- Give sets of 30 compressions and 2 breaths. Each time you give breaths, you need to look in the mouth and remove any object that you see. After removing the object, continue sets of compressions and breaths.
- After 5 sets of 30 compressions and 2 breaths, looking in the mouth (until the object is removed), leave the child to phone 9-1-1 (if not already done) and get an AED.*
- Return to the child or infant and continue CPR. Use the AED as soon as it's available.

*If the small child or infant isn't injured and you're alone, after 5 sets of 30 compressions and 2 breaths, you may carry him with you to phone 9-1-1 and get an AED.

☐ Provide CPR and check for the object in the mouth.
- Give sets of 30 compressions and 2 breaths.
- After each set of 30 compressions, open the airway to give breaths.
- Look in the mouth (Figure 66). If you see an object in the mouth, take it out.
- Give 2 breaths.

☐ Continue providing CPR, checking for the object in the mouth, and using the AED (if available) until you have removed the object.

☐ Then continue providing CPR and using the AED (if available) until
- The child or infant moves, cries, speaks, blinks, or otherwise reacts
- Someone with more advanced training arrives and takes over

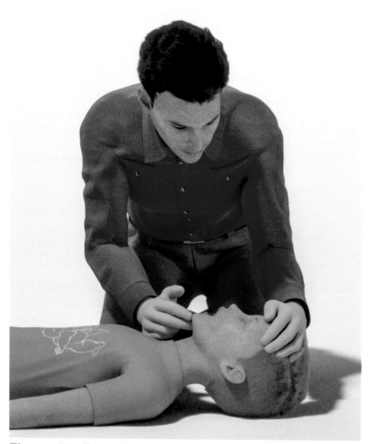

Figure 66. Every time you open the airway to give breaths, look for the object in the back of the throat until the object is removed. Then give 2 breaths.

Conclusion

Summary of High-Quality CPR Components

Component	Adults and Adolescents	Children (Age 1 Year to Puberty)	Infants (Age Less Than 1 Year)
Make sure the scene is safe	Make sure the scene is safe for you and the person needing help		
Tap and shout (check for responsiveness)	Check to see if person is responsive or unresponsive If unresponsive, go to next step		
Shout for help			
Check for breathing	If breathing normally, stay with the person until advanced help arrives If *not* breathing normally or only gasping, begin CPR and use an AED	If breathing, stay with the child or infant until advanced help arrives If *not* breathing or only gasping, begin CPR and use the AED	
Begin CPR, phone 9-1-1, and get an AED	Phone or send someone to phone 9-1-1, begin CPR, and get an AED If you are alone and have a phone, put it on speaker mode and phone 9-1-1 while you begin CPR	Phone or send someone to phone 9-1-1 and get an AED If you are alone and have a phone, put it on speaker mode and phone 9-1-1 while you begin CPR If you are alone and do not have a phone, give 5 sets of 30 compressions and 2 breaths. Then go phone 9-1-1 and get an AED. Return and continue CPR	
Compressions and breaths	30 compressions to 2 breaths		
Compression rate	Push on the chest at a rate of 100 to 120 compressions per minute		
Compression depth	At least 2 inches	At least one third the depth of the chest, or about 2 inches	At least one third the depth of the chest, or about 1½ inches

(continued)

Component	Adults and Adolescents	Children (Age 1 Year to Puberty)	Infants (Age Less Than 1 Year)
Hand placement	2 hands on the lower half of the breastbone	2 hands or 1 hand (optional for very small child) on the lower half of the breastbone	2 fingers in the center of the chest, just below the nipple line
Let the chest come back up	Let the chest come back up to its normal position after each compression		
Interruptions in compressions	Try not to interrupt compressions for more than 10 seconds		

Legal Questions

Good Samaritan laws exist to protect providers who help ill and injured people. The laws vary from state to state. Your instructor will talk to you about the laws that apply to you.

Duty to Provide CPR

Some people may be required to perform CPR while working. Some examples are law enforcement officers, firefighters, flight attendants, lifeguards, and park rangers. If they are off duty, they can choose whether or not to provide CPR.

Providing CPR may be part of your job description. If so, you must help while you're working. However, when you're off duty, you can choose whether to provide CPR.

After the Emergency

If you provide CPR, you may learn private things about a person. You must not share this information with other people. Keep private things private.

Remember to

■ Give all information about the person to EMS rescuers or the person's healthcare providers

■ Protect the person's privacy

After the Heartsaver Pediatric First Aid CPR AED Course

Congratulations on completing this course!

Practice your skills. Review the steps in this workbook often. This will keep you prepared to give first aid care and high-quality CPR whenever it's needed.

It's important to phone 9-1-1 when an emergency arises. The dispatcher will remind you what to do.

Contact the AHA if you want more information on CPR, AEDs, or first aid. You can visit **www.heart.org/cpr** or call 1-877-AHA-4CPR (877-242-4277) to find a class near you.

Even if you don't remember all the steps exactly, it is important for you to try. Any help, even if it isn't perfect, is better than no help at all.

Life Is Why

Science Is Why

Cardiovascular diseases claim more lives than all forms of cancer combined. This unsettling statistic drives the AHA's commitment to bring science to life by advancing resuscitation knowledge and research in new ways.
